MEMORY NOTEBOOK OF NURSING

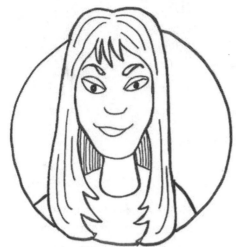

JoAnn Zerwekh, EdD, RN, FNP
Executive Director
Nursing Education Consultants
Ingram, Texas
Nursing Faculty
University of Phoenix
Phoenix, Arizona

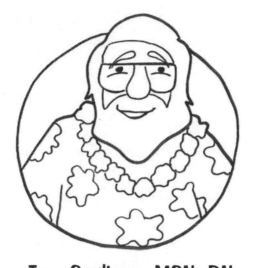

Tom Gaglione, MSN, RN
Nursing Faculty
Kauai Community College
Lihue, Hawaii
Review Course Faculty
Nursing Education Consultants
Ingram, Texas

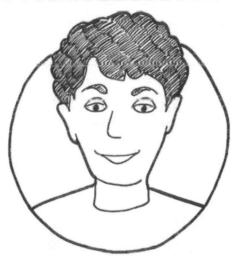

Jo Claborn, MS, RN
Executive Director
Nursing Education Consultants
Ingram, Texas

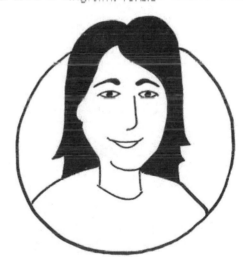

CJ Miller, BSN, RN
Nurse-Illustrator
Washington, Iowa

Artist: C.J. Miller, RN
Washington, Iowa

Production Manager: Mike Cull
Gingerbread Press, Waxahachie, Texas
Desktop Publishing Assistant: James Halfast
San Angelo, Texas

Printed in the United States of America

Nursing Education Consultants
P O Box 465
Ingram, Texas 78025
(800) 933-7277

ISBN 1-892155-07-9
Library of Congress Catalog Number: 2004111861

Any procedure or practice described in this book should be applied by the health-care practitioner under appropriate supervision in accordance with professional standards of care used with regard to the unique circumstances that apply in each practice situation. Care has been taken to confirm the accuracy of information presented and to describe generally accepted practices. However, the authors, editors, and publisher cannot accept any responsibility for errors or omissions or for consequences from application of the information in this book and make no warranty, express or implied, with respect to the contents of this book.

This book is written to be used as a study aid and review book for nursing. It is not intended for use as a primary resource for procedures, treatments, medications or to serve as a complete textbook for nursing care. Copies of this book may be obtained directly from Nursing Education Consultants.

Last Digit is the Print Number: 4 3 2 1

Preface

The *Memory Notebook of Nursing: Pharmacology & Diagnostic Tests* is a new and different approach for us. We have listened to you and your enthusiastic responses and chose to create this next *Memory Notebook of Nursing* with a more focused approach on the areas of Pharmacology and Diagnostic Tests. As always, we continue our proven use of accelerated learning tools. We are excited to introduce the creative and humorous mind of Tom Gaglione, RN, MSN, nurse educator, and one of our own Nursing Education Consultant's faculty and frequent presenter on the humor of "Surviving Nursing School," who has teamed up with our own creative and talented artist and nurse, C.J. Miller. We are pleased to bring this new volume to you and hope that it helps you to learn new concepts, expand your knowledge base, and at times just laugh out loud at the fun of it, as we found ourselves doing during its creation.

To assist you in the utilization of this book, here is a little information about accelerated learning and how you can enhance your learning by utilizing both the left (analytical, linear, logical, rote memory) side of your brain and the right (visual, images, musical, imaginative) side of your brain. Several techniques are used to encourage the whole-brain to think and learn concepts. These techniques are memory tools and mnemonics. Memory tools are aids to assist you to draw associations from other ideas with the use of visual images to help cement the learning. Mnemonics are most often words, phrases, or sentences that help you remember information. Throughout this book, you will find ideas that we have found useful in teaching students how to remember information. As you read over each illustration, get involved with the process and write down your own ideas on the drawings. Think about this, color activates the brain and music increases right brain activity. As you are coloring or writing, turn on some music (no words or singing just instrumental music), don't be afraid to experiment and find out what type of music works for you!

We hope you enjoy this new addition to our *Memory Notebook of Nursing* series.

Good health, happiness, and success in your future!

JoAnn Zerwekh

Jo Carol Claborn

Acknowledgments

We really have you, the students and faculty, to thank for the creation of this new edition to our series. It was the continuous "Battle Cry" of "When is the next *Memory Notebook of Nursing* coming out?" We heard it from students and faculty at nursing conventions and during our review courses held around the country. We are very pleased to bring this new work to all who have been so supportive of this endeavor.

I want to thank my partner and boss, JoAnn Zerwekh, for her trust, support, and love while giving birth to this brain child. I'm sure she wants to thank me for taking the initiative in its creation and allowing her and her incredible editorial skills to proof my work before unleashing it on the public.

I, also would like thank my other boss and friend, Jo Carol Clabon, for her faith and trust by allowing me the opportunity to add to the series of their incredibly successful *Memory Notebooks of Nursing*.

Jo Carol and JoAnn (both nurses) over the past 25 years have worked to help tens of thousands of student nurses through their publications and review courses to fulfill their dream of becoming professional registered nurses.

I want thank C.J. Miller, nurse and artist, whose incredible artistic gift gave form to my characters and thoughts. Without you, my creation would still be just a thought. I also want to thank your husband, Jeff, for his kindness on the phone and always knowing where I could find you when I called.

And of course. Jo Carol's husband, Robert, my partner in crime when we are all together. Thank you for always being there for all of us. "You be the Man!"

Dedication

I dedicate this book to the most creative woman I know, my Mother Carmella Gaglione, who always put the family first no matter where in the world we lived. You have always been there for me through the hardest of times. My heart and love are always with you Mom.

Tom Gaglione, RN, MSN

Table of Contents

Aminoglycosides

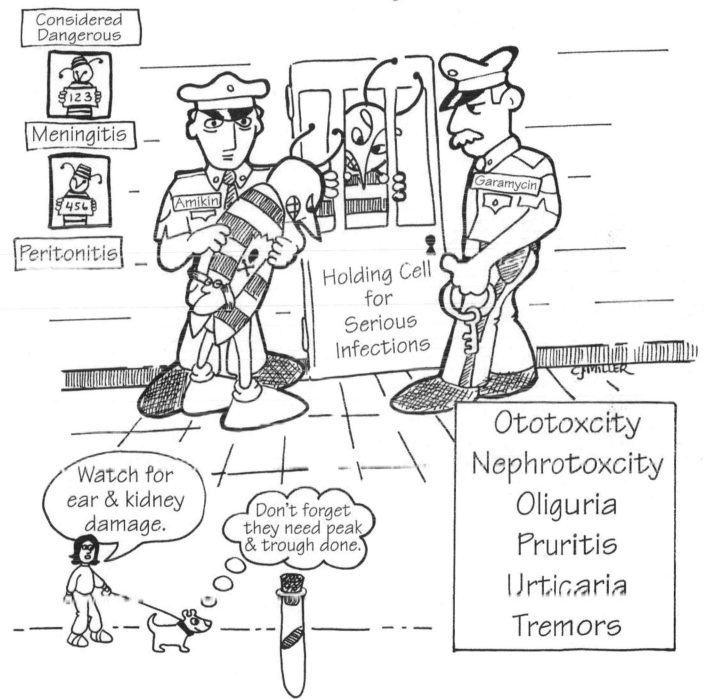

Aminoglycosides - Serum Peak and Trough

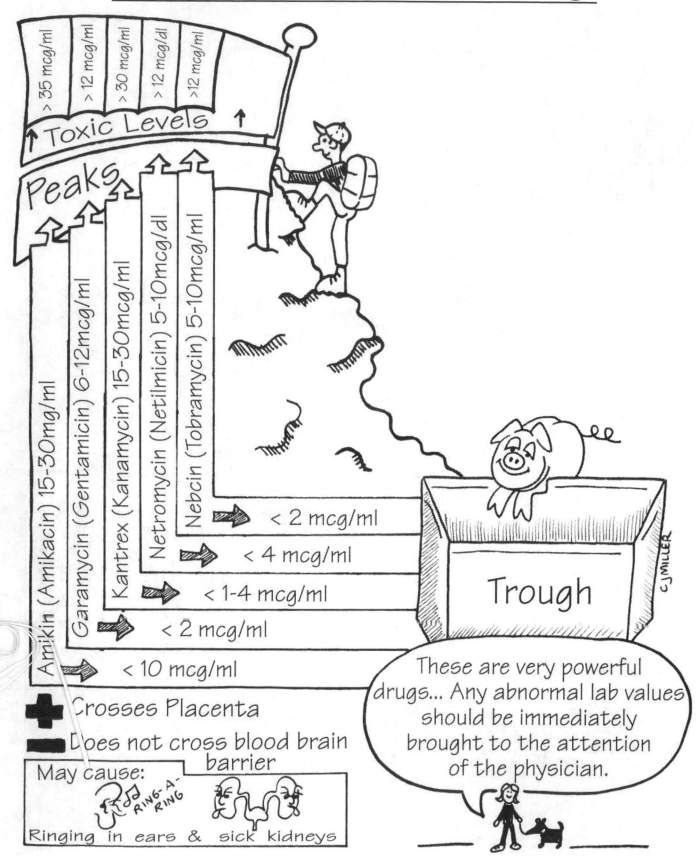

Toxic Levels

> 35 mcg/ml
> 12 mcg/ml
> 30 mcg/dl
> 12 mcg/dl
>12 mcg/ml

Peaks

Amikin (Amikacin) 15-30mg/ml
Garamycin (Gentamicin) 6-12mcg/ml
Kantrex (Kanamycin) 15-30mcg/ml
Netromycin (Netilmicin) 5-10mcg/dl
Nebcin (Tobramycin) 5-10mcg/ml

< 2 mcg/ml
< 4 mcg/ml
< 1-4 mcg/ml
< 2 mcg/ml
< 10 mcg/ml

Trough

+ Crosses Placenta

– Does not cross blood brain barrier

May cause:
RING-A-RING
Ringing in ears & sick kidneys

These are very powerful drugs... Any abnormal lab values should be immediately brought to the attention of the physician.

Antibiotics/Antivirals
Memory Notebook of Nursing: Pharmacology & Diagnostics

© 2005 Nursing Education
Consultants, Inc.

Amoxicillin (Amoxil)

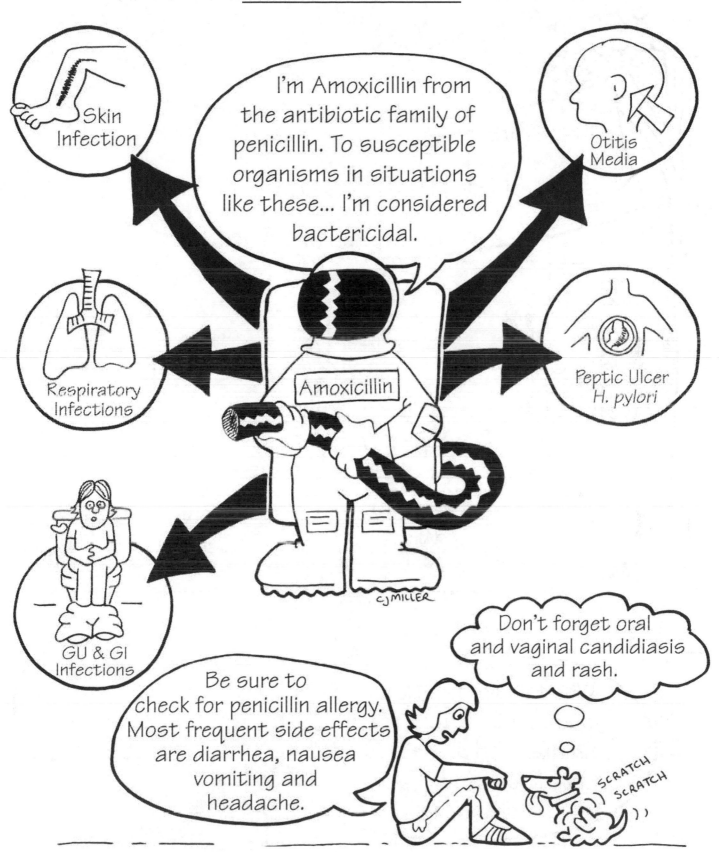

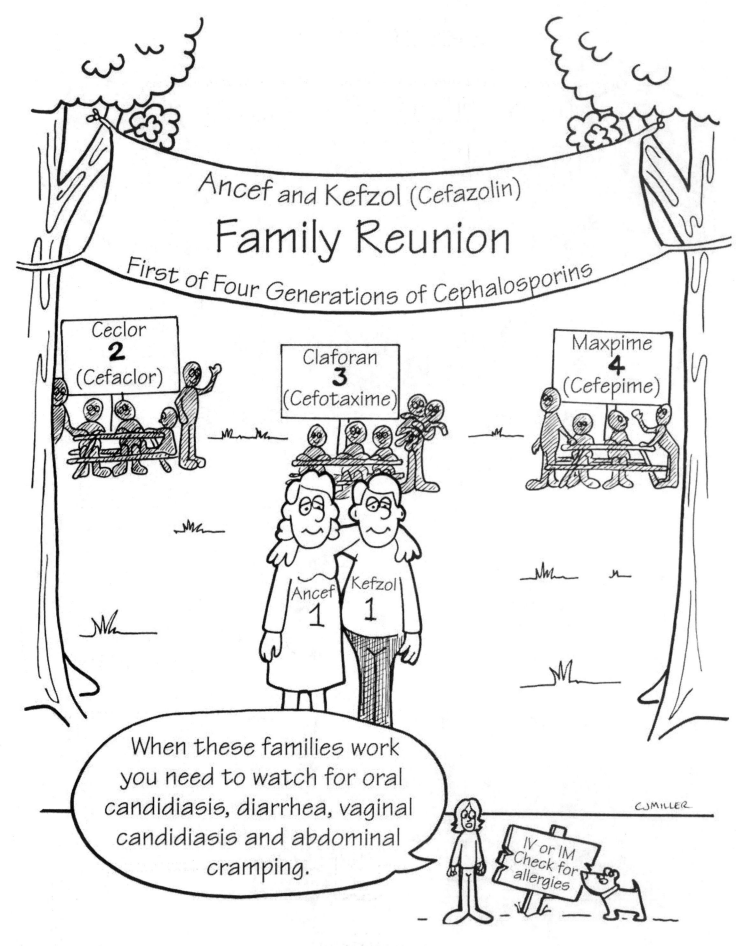

Antiretrovirals

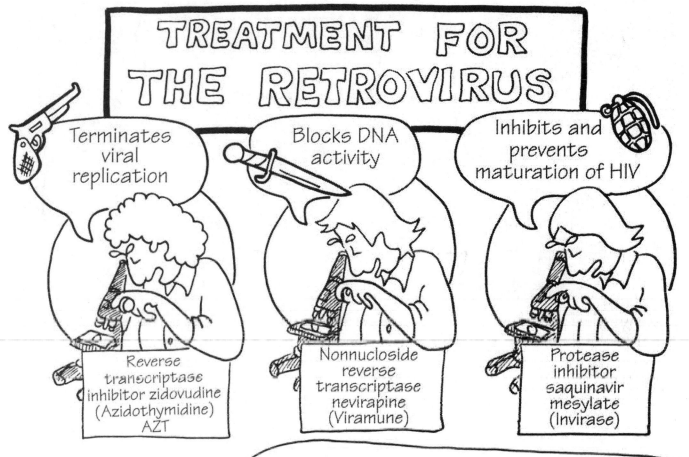

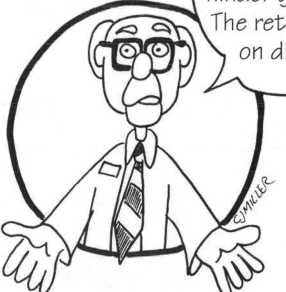

Cephalosporins

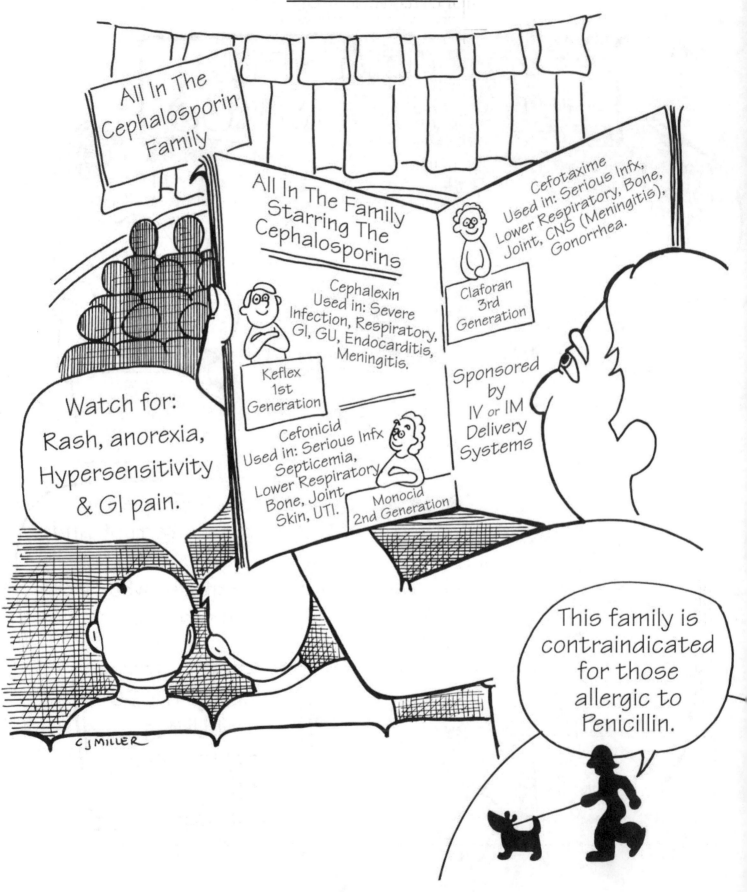

Antibiotics/Antivirals
Memory Notebook of Nursing: Pharmacology & Diagnostics

© 2005 Nursing Education
Consultants, Inc.

Ciprofloxacin (Cipro)

"For those hard to reach chronic bacterial infections"

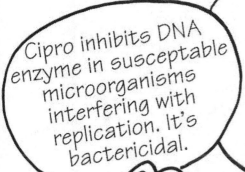

Cipro inhibits DNA enzyme in susceptable microorganisms interfering with replication. It's bactericidal.

Cipro is used to treat bacterial infections in the urinary, respiratory & GI tract as well as with bone, joint and ophthalmic infections.

Caution should be taken with renal or cns disorders, seizures or those taking Theophylline or caffeine.

WARNING:

Can cause nausea, diarrhea, dyspepsia, vomiting, constipation, flatulence and confusion.

Toxic effects can cause superinfection (enteroccal or fungal).

Assess the client for hypersensitivity history. Be sure the client knows to take all the prescribed doses and to increase fluid intake during therapy.

It can also cause headache, dizziness, restlessness and seizures.

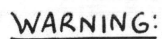

Metronidazole (Flagyl)

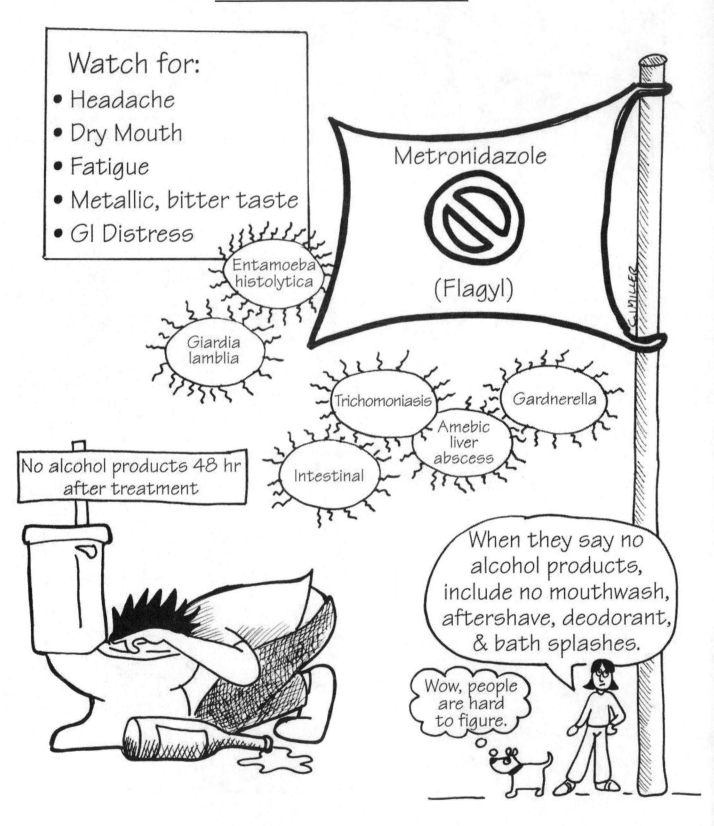

Isoniazid (INH)

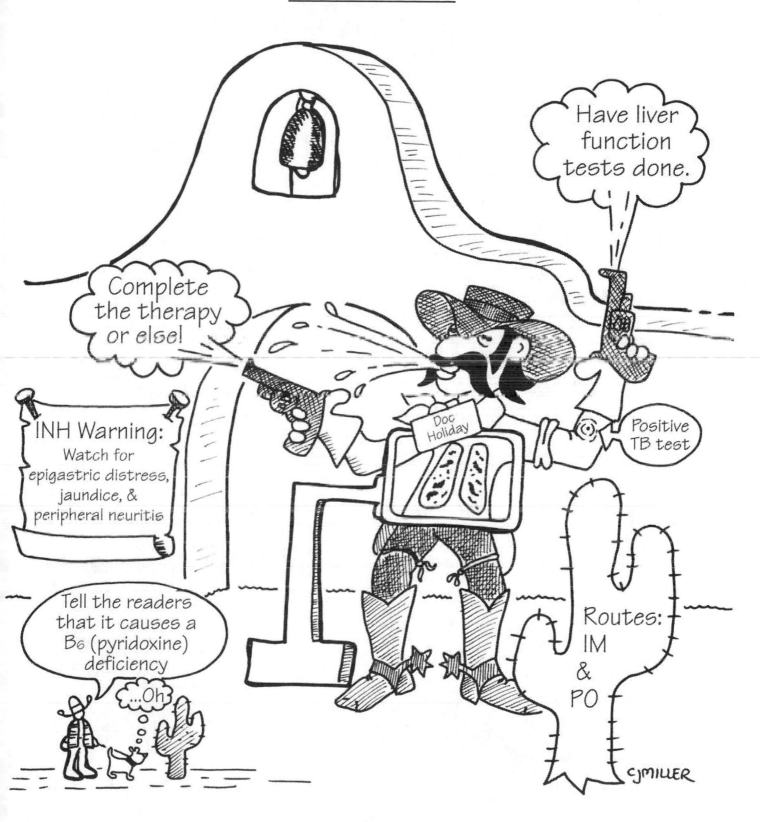

Clotrimazole (Lotrimin)

"One Way to Say No to Yeast!"

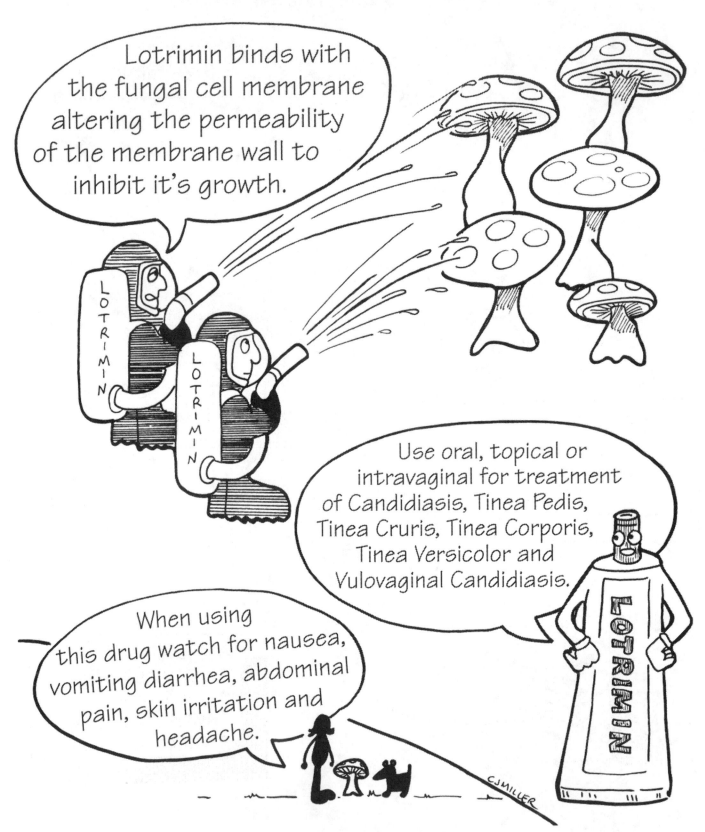

Antibiotics/Antivirals
Memory Notebook of Nursing: Pharmacology & Diagnostics

© 2005 Nursing Education
Consultants, Inc.

Tequin (Gatifloxacin)

"Tequin for Acute Bacterial Exacerbations"

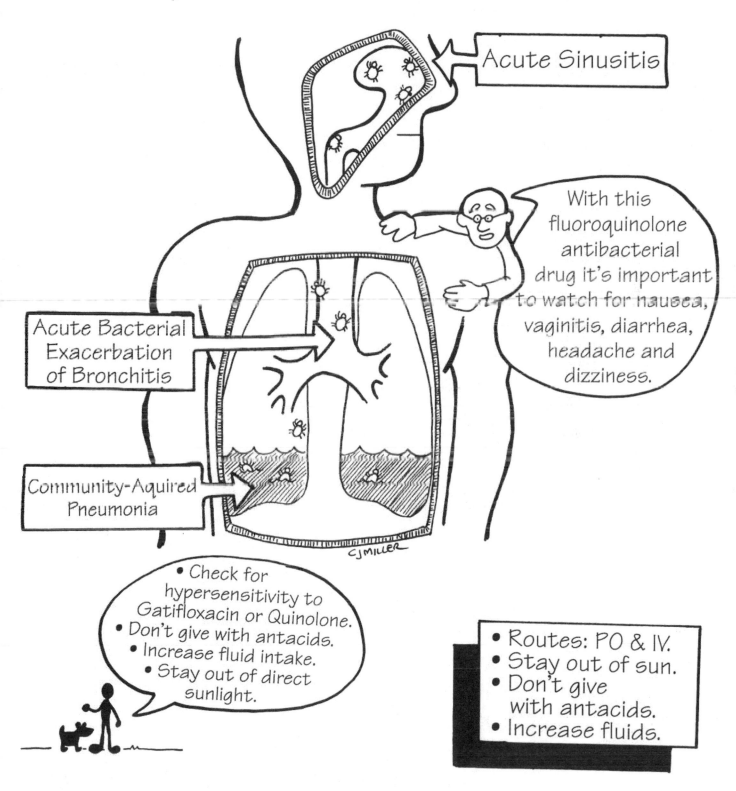

Tetracycline Uses

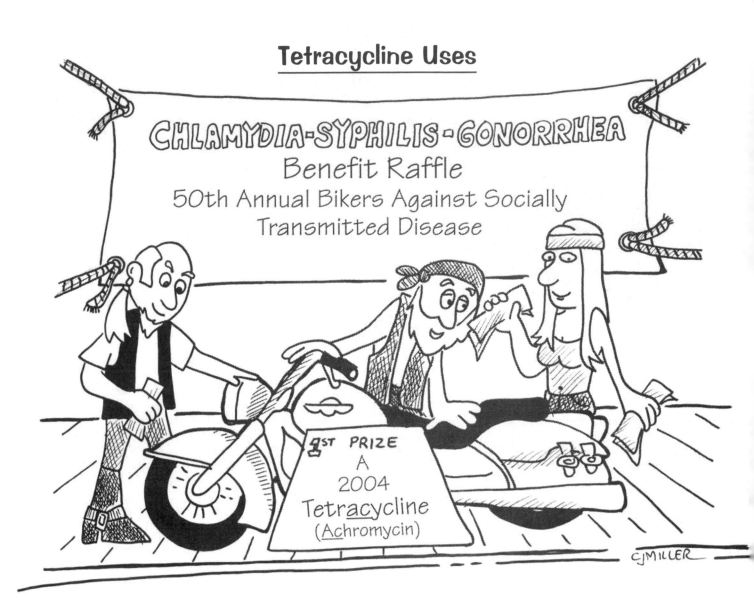

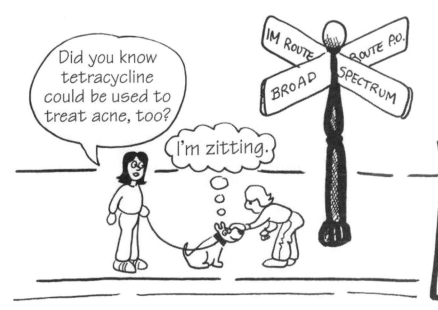

Watch for:
- Epigastric discomfort
- Diarrhea
- Heartburn
- Photosensitivity

Antibiotics/Antivirals
Memory Notebook of Nursing: Pharmacology & Diagnostics

Respigam

Respiratory Syncytial Virus Immune Globulin

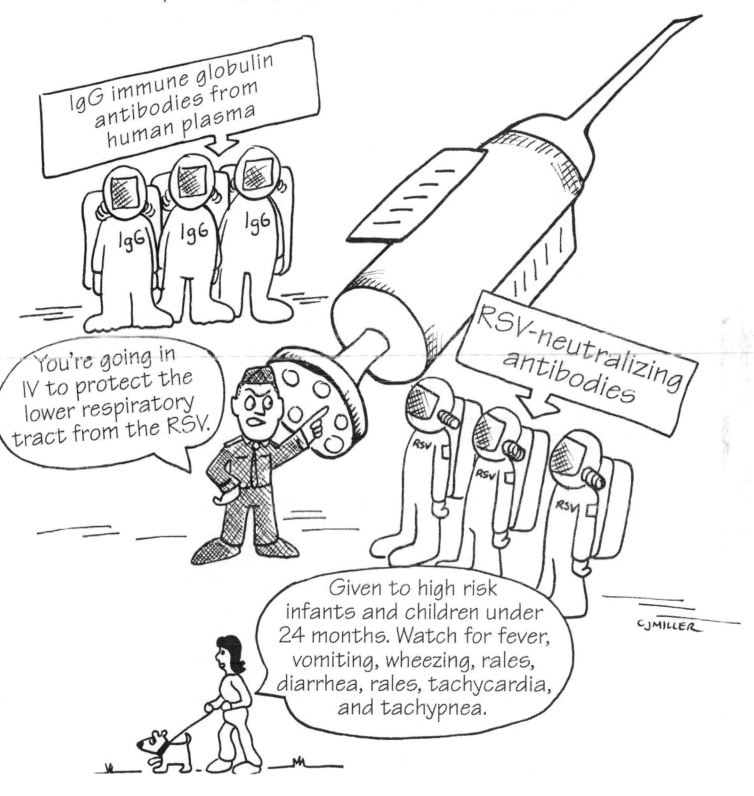

Rocephin

"IV or IM, Rocephin (Ceftriaxone) Does the Job Against Bacterial Infections"

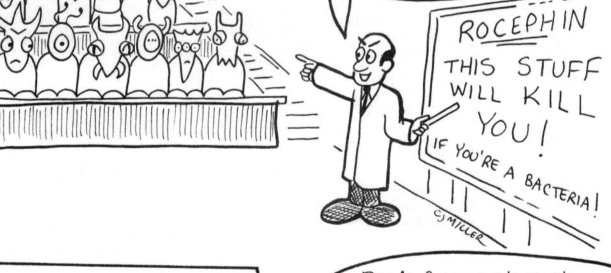

For those of you attacking the respiratory and GI tract, or causing acute bacterial otitis media or septicemia, you're going to have the fight of your life!

ROCEPHIN THIS STUFF WILL KILL YOU! IF YOU'RE A BACTERIA!

CJ MILLER

Toxic: colitis, superinfections and nephrotoxicity. Can be given IV or IM. Either way can cause oral or vaginal candidiasis, diarrhea and abdominal cramping.

Don't forget that the IM injection is painful and may cause nausea and serum sickness reaction. Ask your client about any allergic reactions to Cephalosporins or Penicillins.

Azithromycin (Zithromax)

Top to Bottom... Mild to Moderate

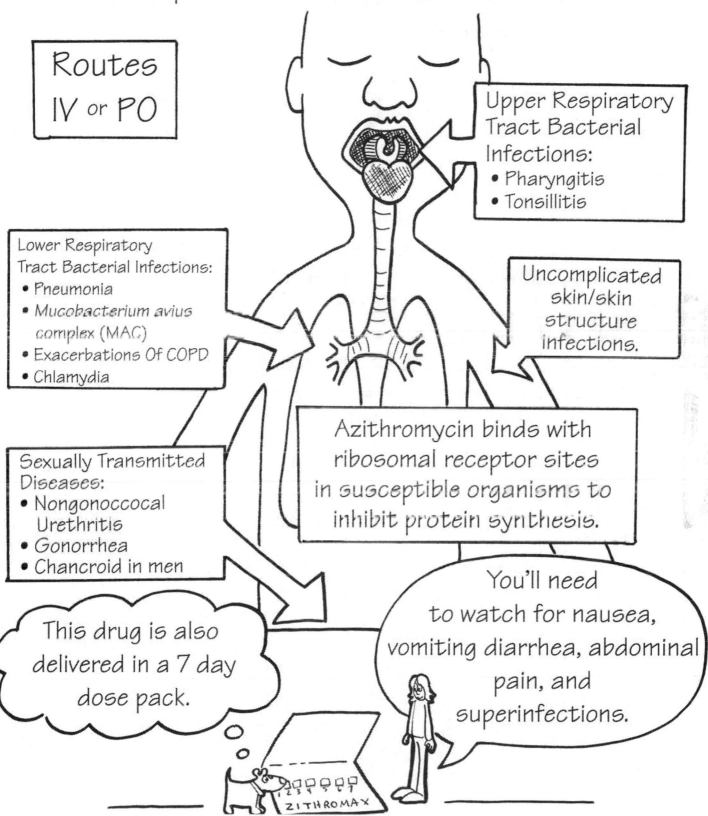

Routes
IV or PO

Upper Respiratory Tract Bacterial Infections:
• Pharyngitis
• Tonsillitis

Lower Respiratory Tract Bacterial Infections:
• Pneumonia
• Mucobacterium avius complex (MAC)
• Exacerbations Of COPD
• Chlamydia

Uncomplicated skin/skin structure infections.

Azithromycin binds with ribosomal receptor sites in susceptible organisms to inhibit protein synthesis.

Sexually Transmitted Diseases:
• Nongonoccocal Urethritis
• Gonorrhea
• Chancroid in men

This drug is also delivered in a 7 day dose pack.

You'll need to watch for nausea, vomiting diarrhea, abdominal pain, and superinfections.

ZITHROMAX

Leukeran (Chlorambucil)

"Abnormal cell growth called Lymphocytic Leukemia, Non-Hodgkin's and Hodgkin's Disease"

Leukeran is an alkylating agent that kills by the alkyalation of cell DNA.

Extreme caution should be used within one month of a full-course of radiation therapy or myelosuppressive drug therapy.

As with any anti-neoplastic drug... watch for GI effects (nausea, vomiting, anorexia and diarrhea), as well as alopecia. The real problem will be bone marrow depression reflected in hematologic toxicity.

Bones can be depressed?

A CBC should be performed each week during therapy, WBC every 3-6 weeks of therapy.

Antineoplastic
Memory Notebook of Nursing: Pharmacology & Diagnostics

ACE Inhibitors

Antiotensin - Converting Enzyme

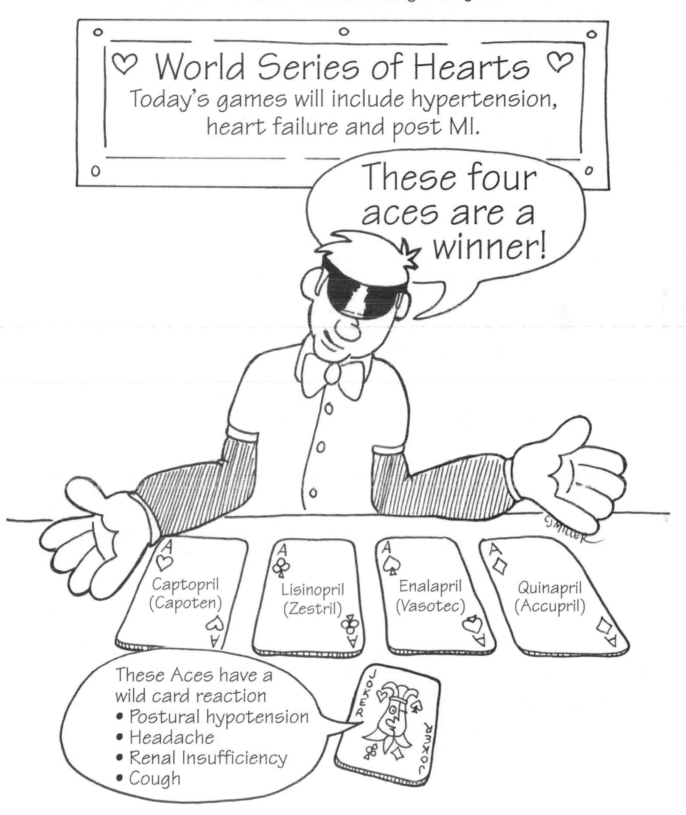

Antiarryhthmics

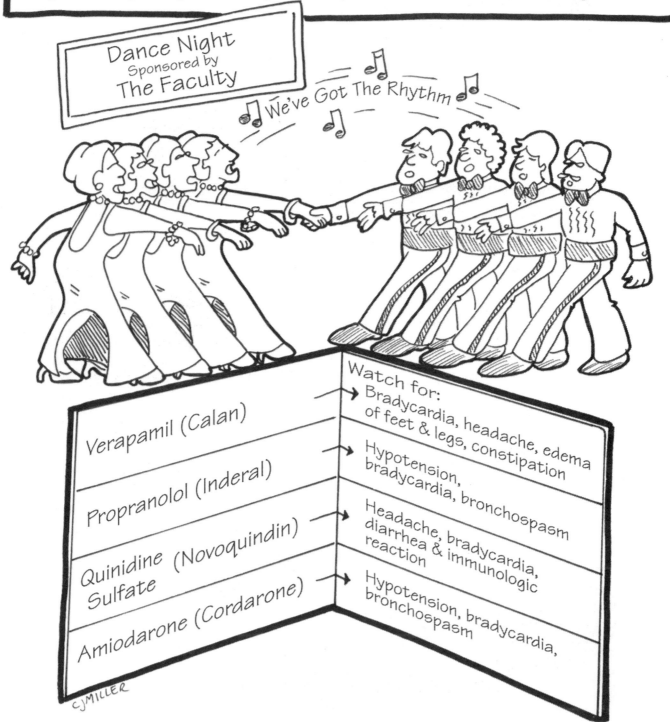

THE ANTIARRHYTHMIC SCHOOL OF DANCE

If you've got good rhythm, you can dance to any beat

Dance Night
Sponsored by
The Faculty

♪ We've Got The Rhythm ♪

	Watch for:
Verapamil (Calan)	Bradycardia, headache, edema of feet & legs, constipation
Propranolol (Inderal)	Hypotension, bradycardia, bronchospasm
Quinidine (Novoquindin) Sulfate	Headache, bradycardia, diarrhea & immunologic reaction
Amiodarone (Cordarone)	Hypotension, bradycardia, bronchospasm,

CJMILLER

Cardiac
Memory Notebook of Nursing: Pharmacology & Diagnostics

Antihypertensives

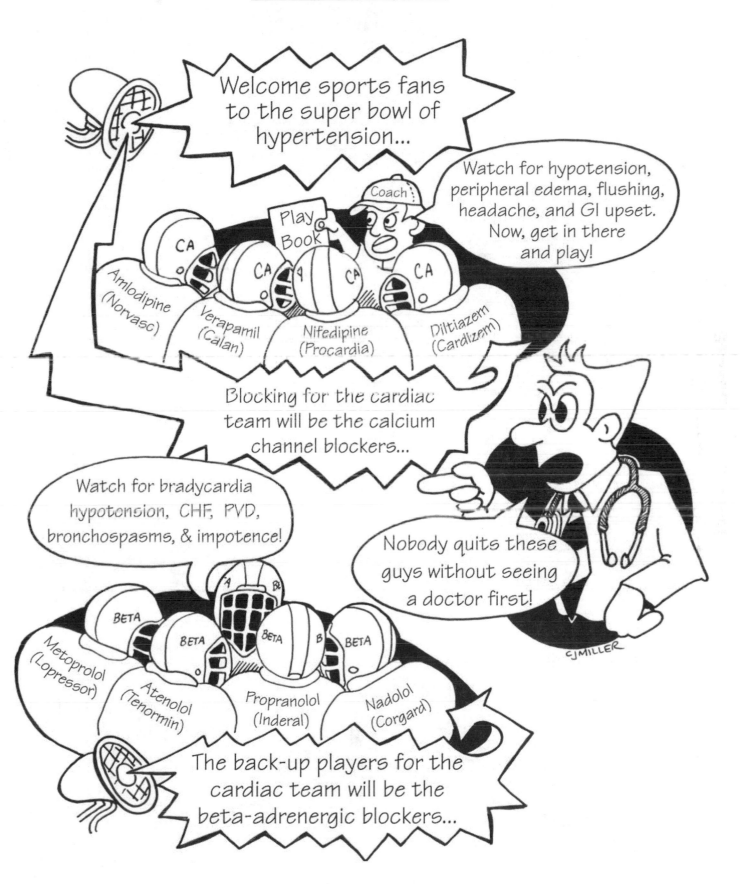

Cordarone (Amiodarone)

"Don Cordarone... The Enforcer"

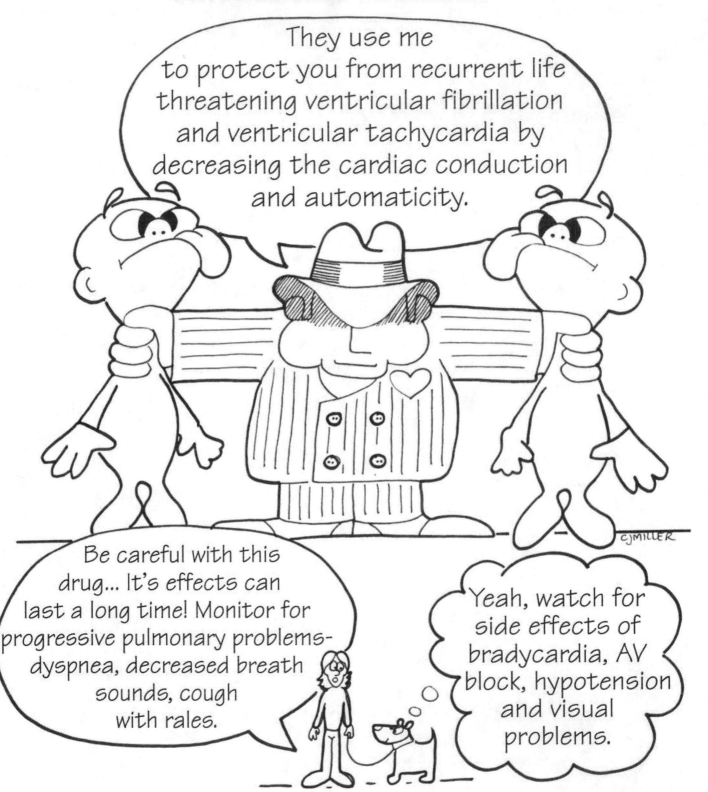

Cardiac
Memory Notebook of Nursing: Pharmacology & Diagnostics

The Wizard of Digitalis

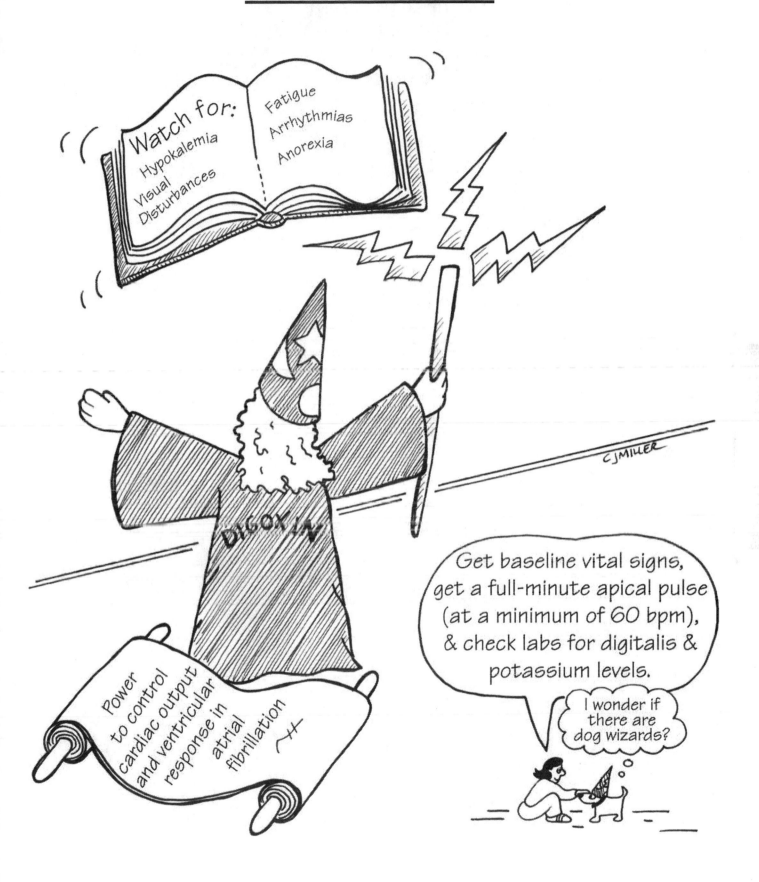

Fosinopril (Monopril)

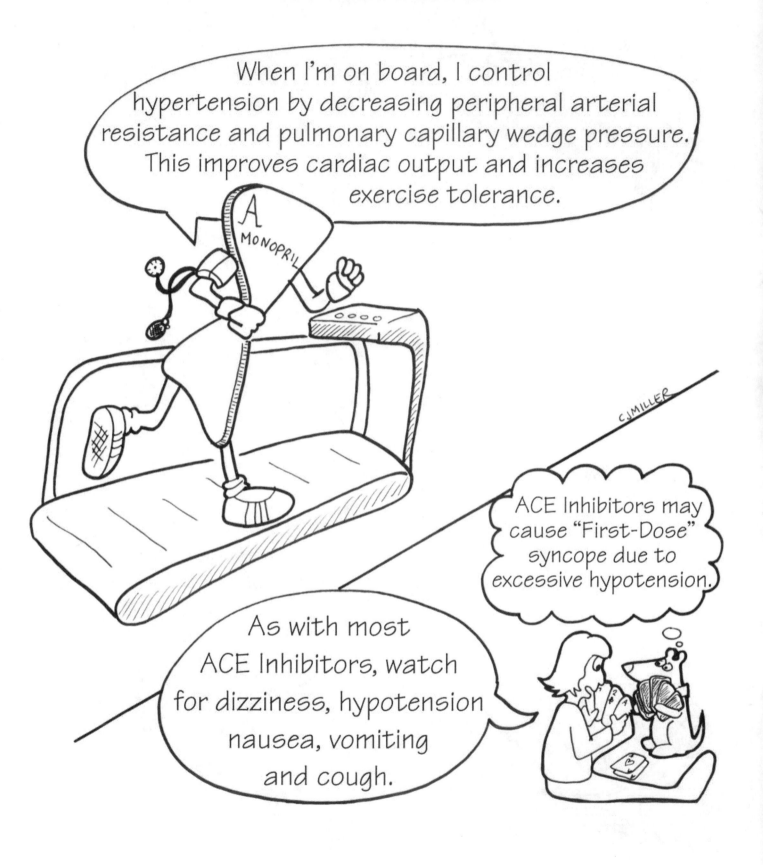

Nitroglycerin

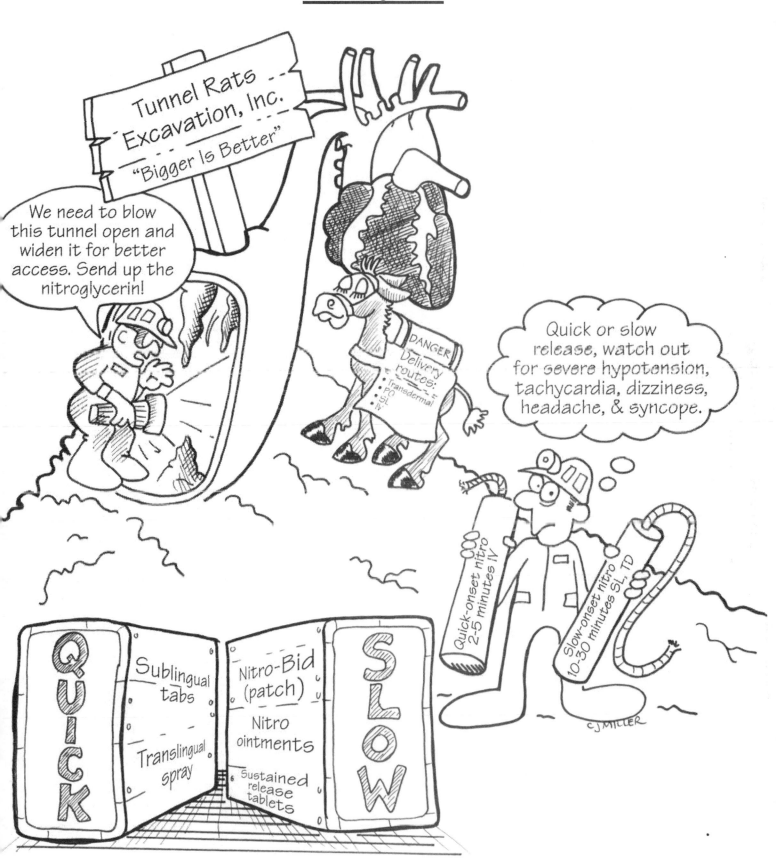

Antihistamines

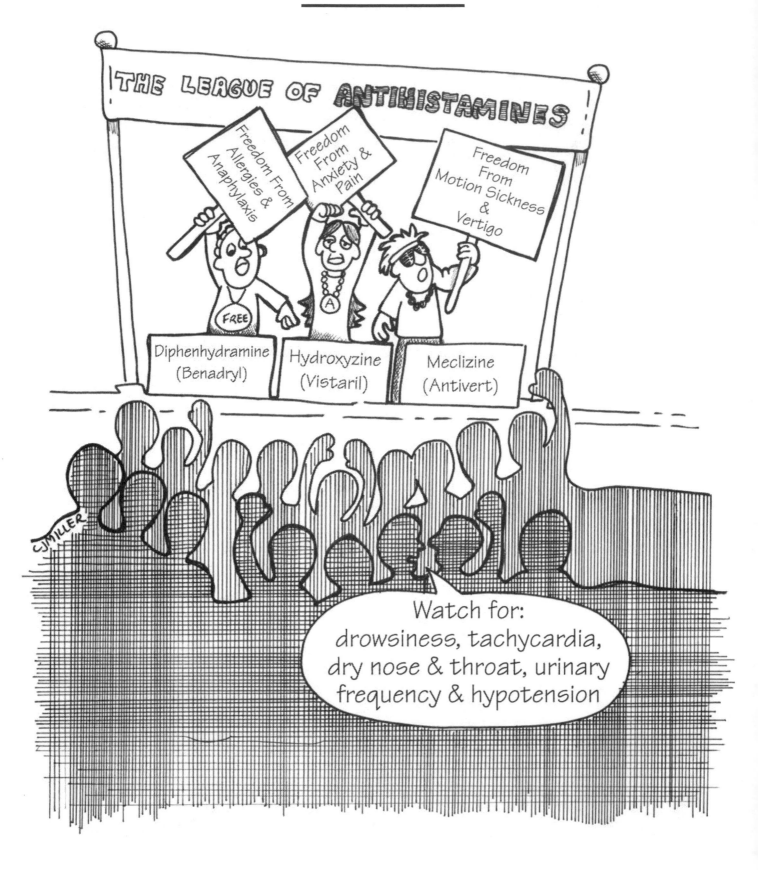

Antitussives, Expectorants & Mucolytics

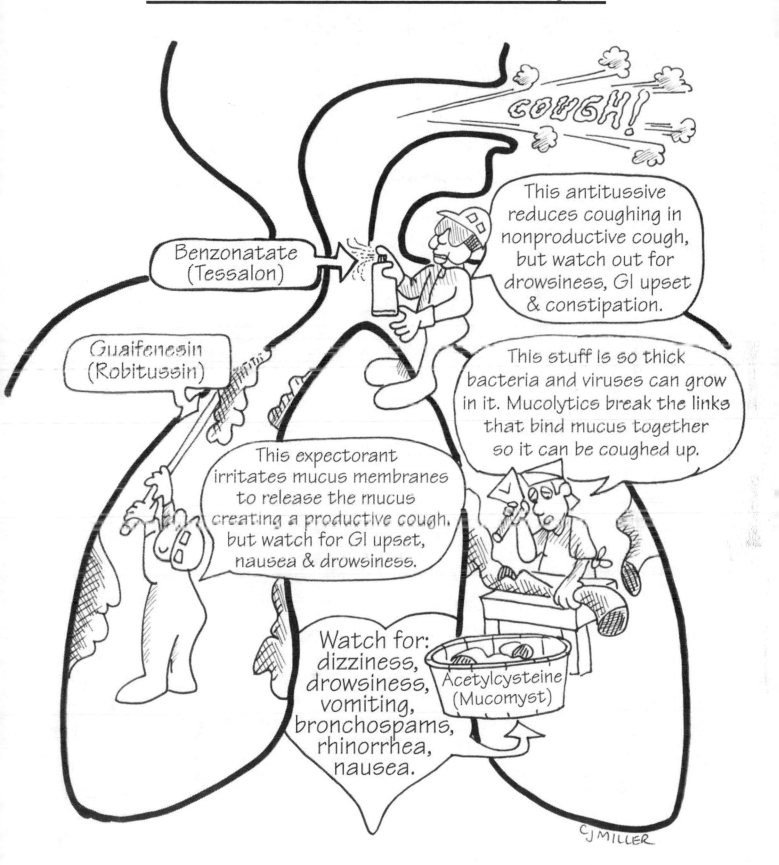

Bronchodilators

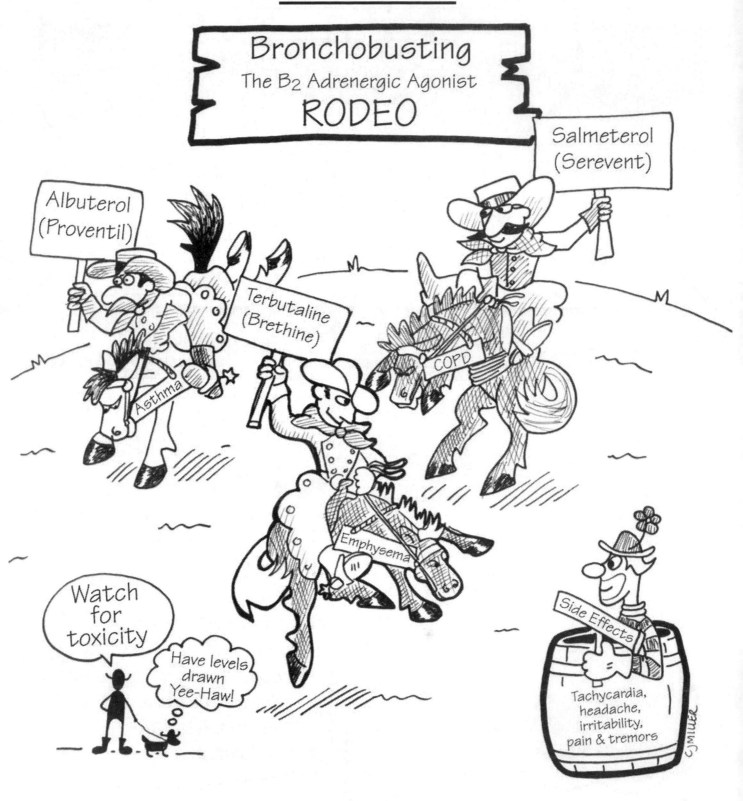

Pulmicort (Budesonide)

"It's a Matter of Life and Breath"

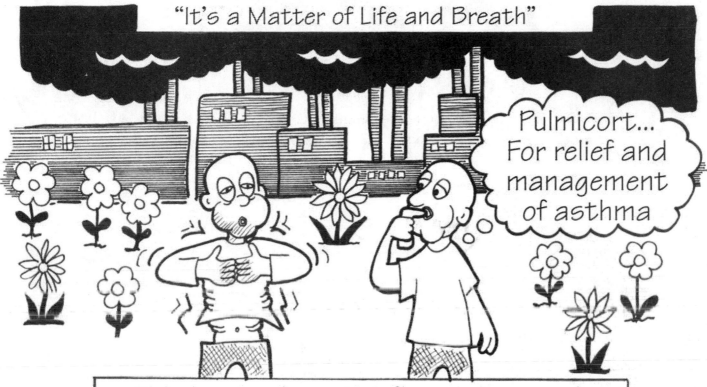

© 2005 Nursing Education Consultants, Inc.

Cetirizine (Zyrtec)

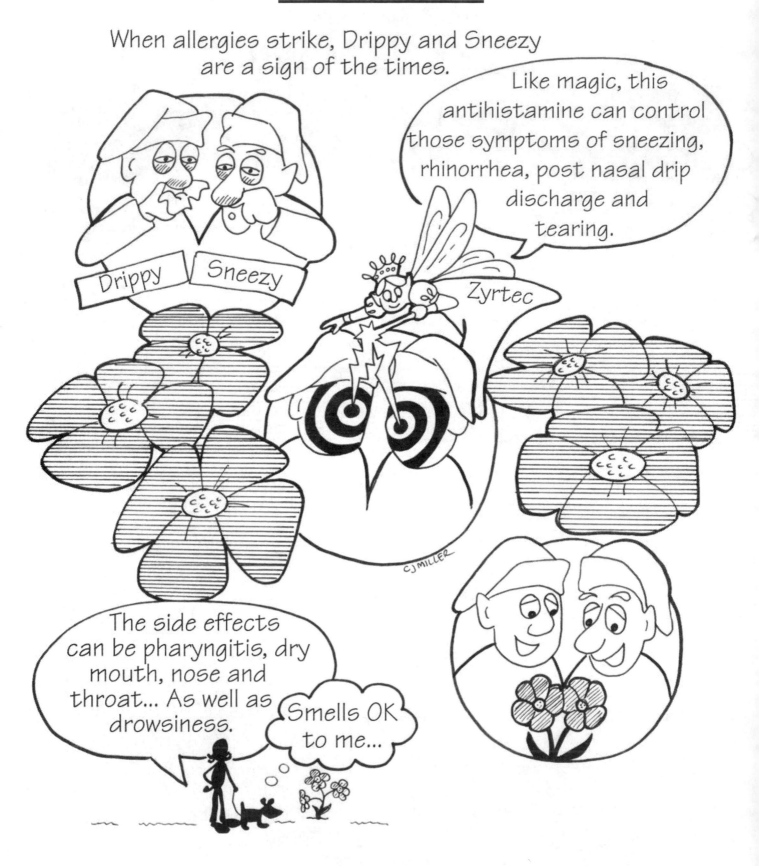

Antidiarrheals

Loperamide (Imodium) and
Diphenoxylate Hydrocholride (Lomotil)
- With Atropine Sulfate -

Gotta Go, Gotta Go, Gotta Go, Go Go!

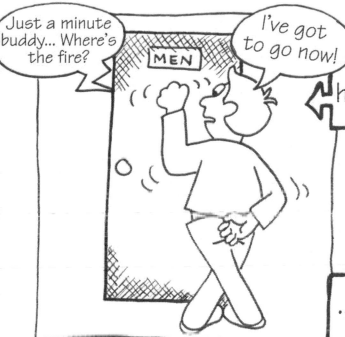

Just a minute buddy... Where's the fire?

MEN

I've got to go now!

Does diarrhea always seem to hit when you are out on the town...

...When mother nature calls... Is it the wrong number???

...It's time to take control with Imodium & Lomotil.

Watch for sedation, flushing, tachycardia, fatigue, depression, GI discomfort & constipation.

I poop in the woods.

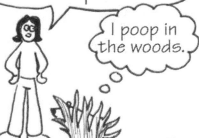

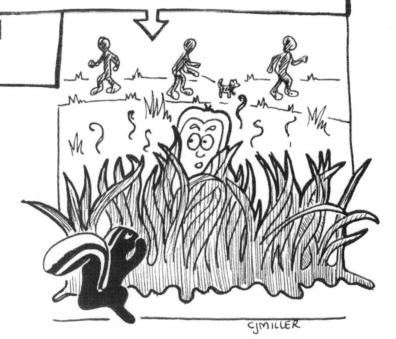

CJMILLER

Memory Notebook of Nursing: Pharmacology & Diagnostics

Amphojel (Aluminum Hydroxide)

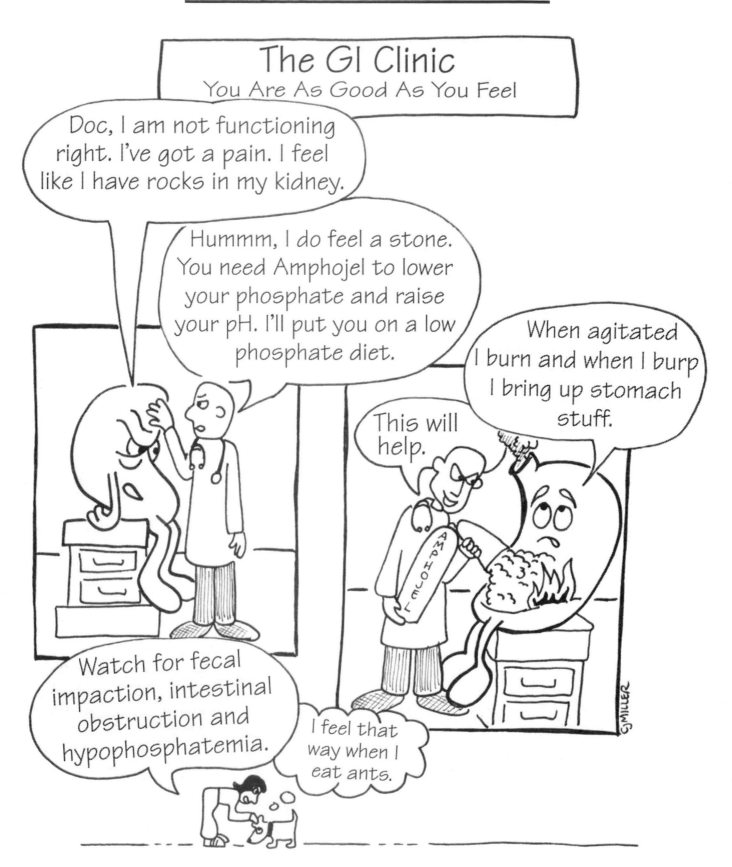

Prochlorperazine (Compazine)

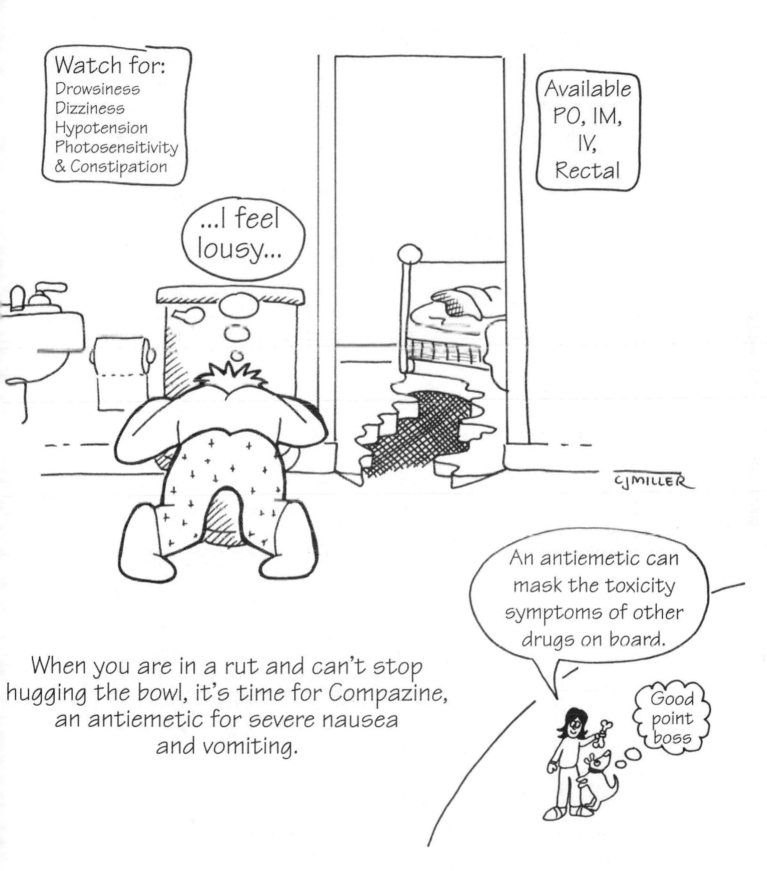

Memory Notebook of Nursing: Pharmacology & Diagnostics

Bisacodyl (Ducolax)

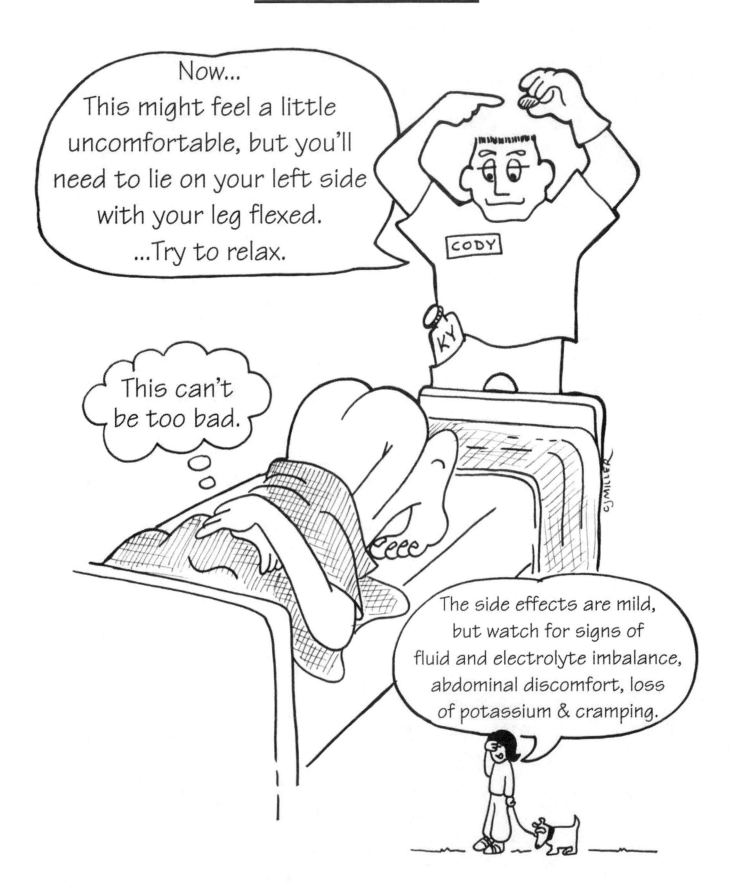

Kayexalate

(Sodium Polystyrene Sulfonate)

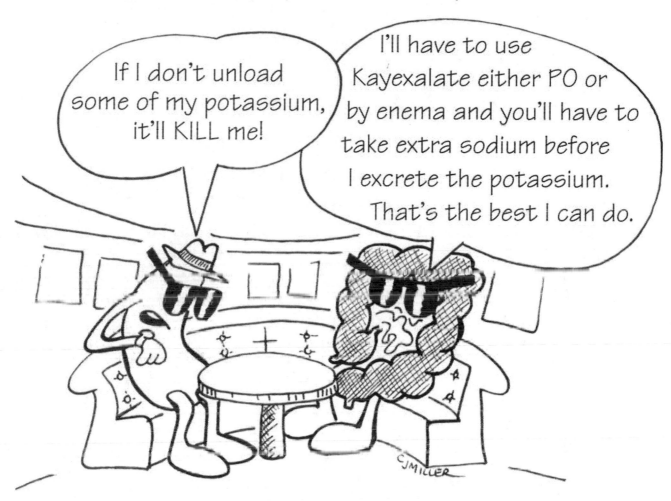

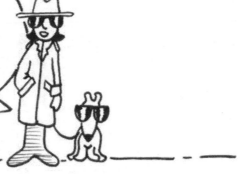

Lactulose

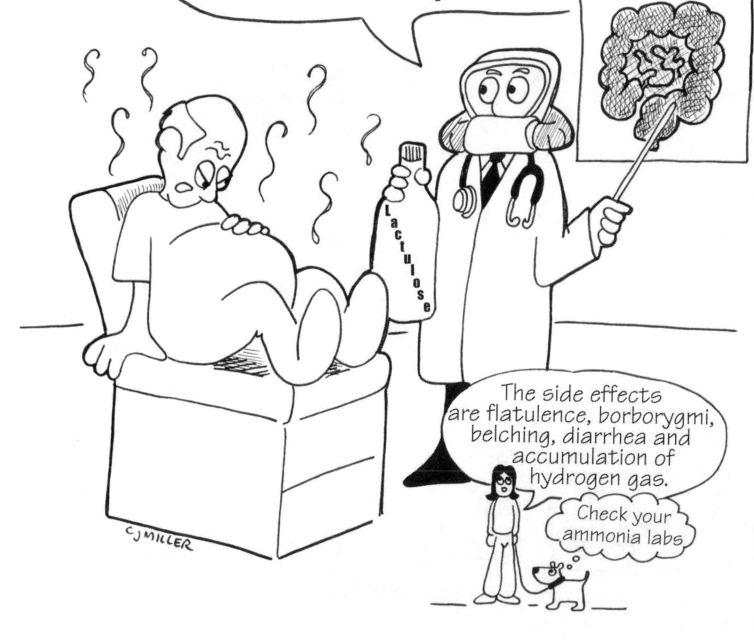

Gemfibrozil (Lopid)

"If it tastes good, it's probably bad for you."

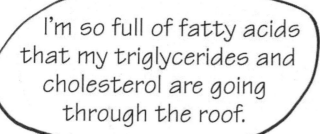

I'm so full of fatty acids that my triglycerides and cholesterol are going through the roof.

I'm going to help decrease your uptake of fatty acids, this will help decrease serum triglycerides and very low density lipoproteins (VDLD).

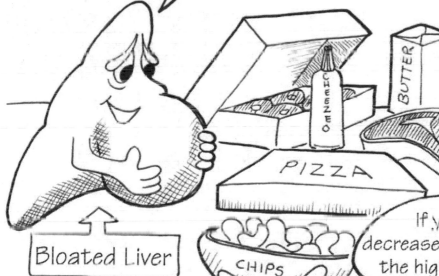

Bloated Liver

CHEEZEO

BUTTER

PIZZA

CHIPS

If you let lopid help, he'll decrease your VDLD's and increase the high density lipoproteins (HDL's).

You need to watch those liver enzymes for signs of muscle tenderness, pain, gallstones, dyspepsia, diarrhea, nausea and vomiting.

I need this stuff when I eat ice cream.

Psyllium (Metamucil)

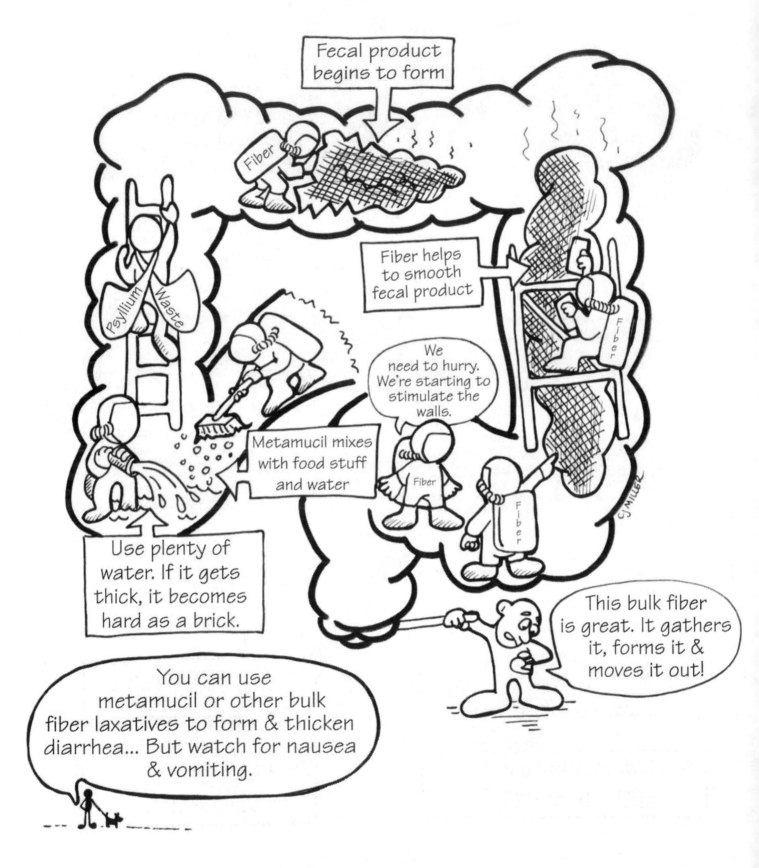

GI
Memory Notebook of Nursing: Pharmacology & Diagnostics

Magnesium Hydroxide (Milk of Magnesia)

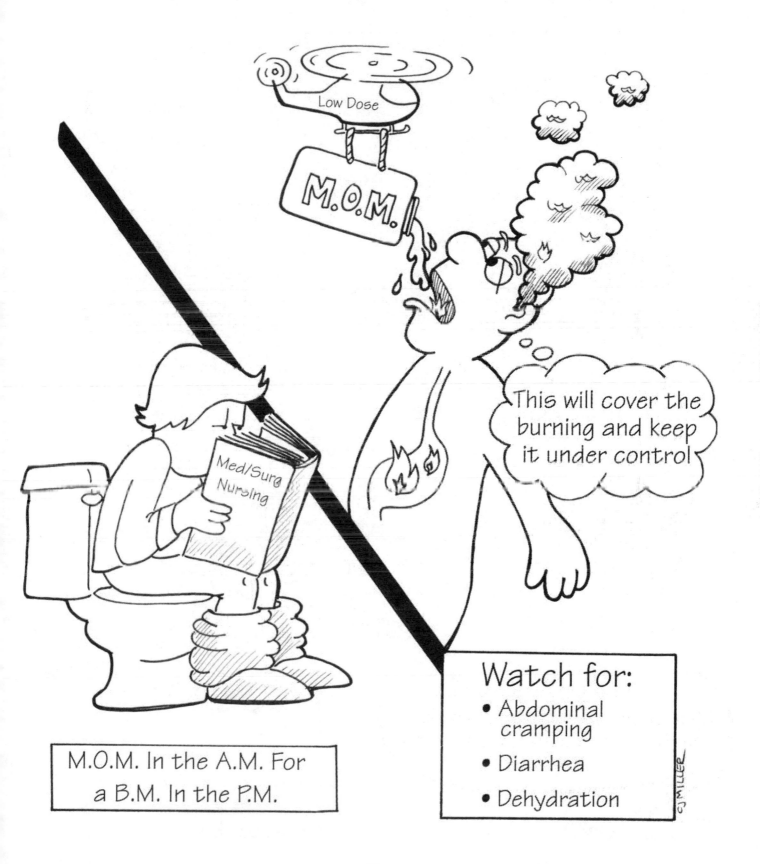

M.O.M. In the A.M. For a B.M. In the P.M.

Watch for:
- Abdominal cramping
- Diarrhea
- Dehydration

Memory Notebook of Nursing: Pharmacology & Diagnostics

Promethazine (Phenergan)

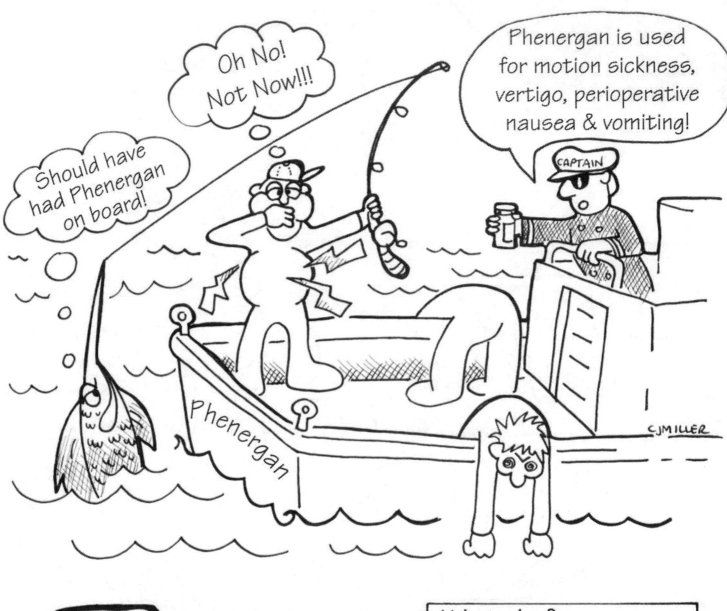

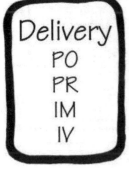

Delivery
PO
PR
IM
IV

Watch for:
- Drowsiness
- Restlessness
- Hypo or Hypertension
- Constipation

Omeprazole (Prilosec)

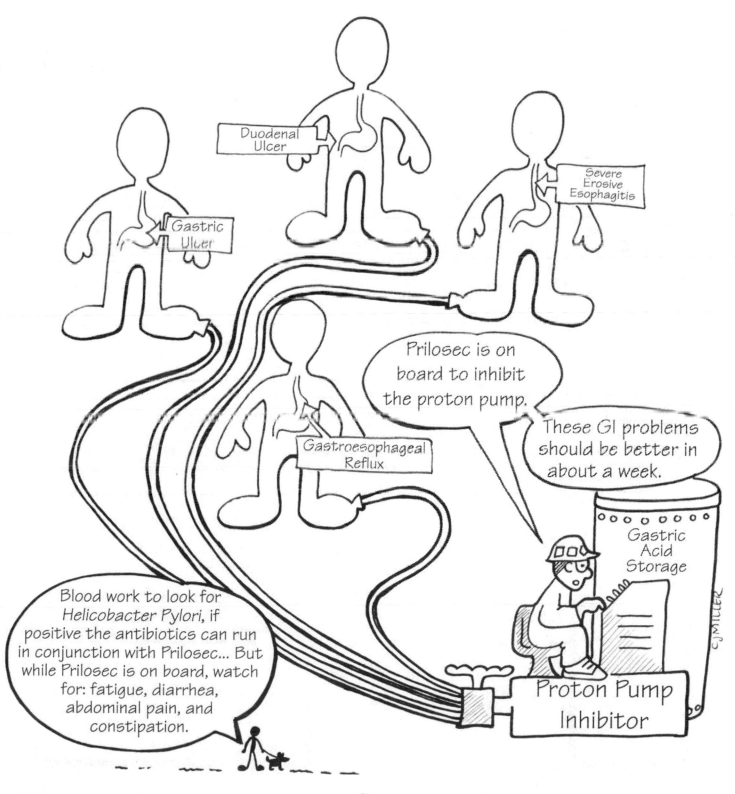

Cholestyramine Resin (Questran)

"Separating the Good From the Bad"

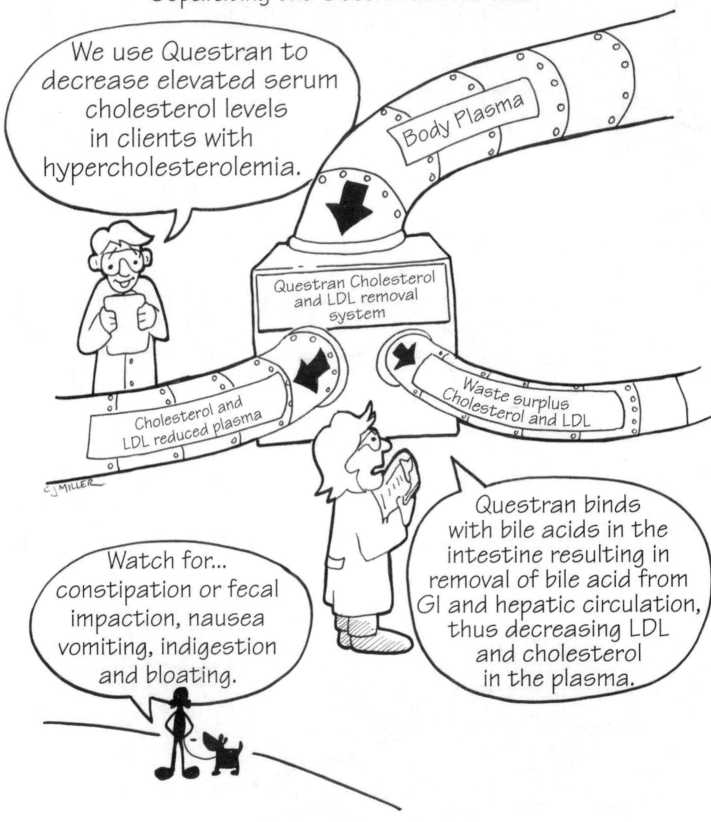

GI
Memory Notebook of Nursing: Pharmacology & Diagnostics

Metoclopramide (Reglan)

Welcome to Jamaica!
The Annual Prokinetic Agent Convention

Ya mon, Reglan be making the smooth muscles move so the tract be all right!

Watch out for sedation, insomnia diarrhea and constipation.

Rasta Dog

Used in treatment of delayed gastric emptying & GERD.

Ranitidine (Zantac) and Cimetidine (Tagamet)

The Wrestling Federation Presents
H2 Receptor Antagonist Smack Down!

Zantac &
Tagamet

Painful Duodenal Ulcer
& Burny Gastroesophageal
Reflux

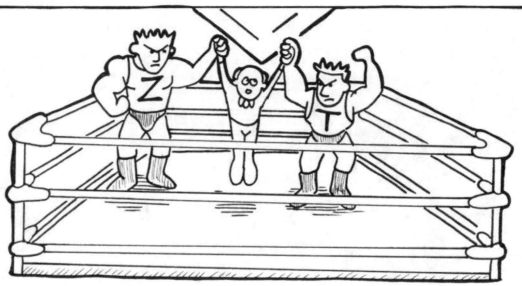

All proceeds will go for the reduction
of basal gastric acid release.

CJ MILLER

Watch for:
• Headache
• Diarrhea
• Depression
• GI Disturbances
• Rash

Spironolactone (Aldactone)

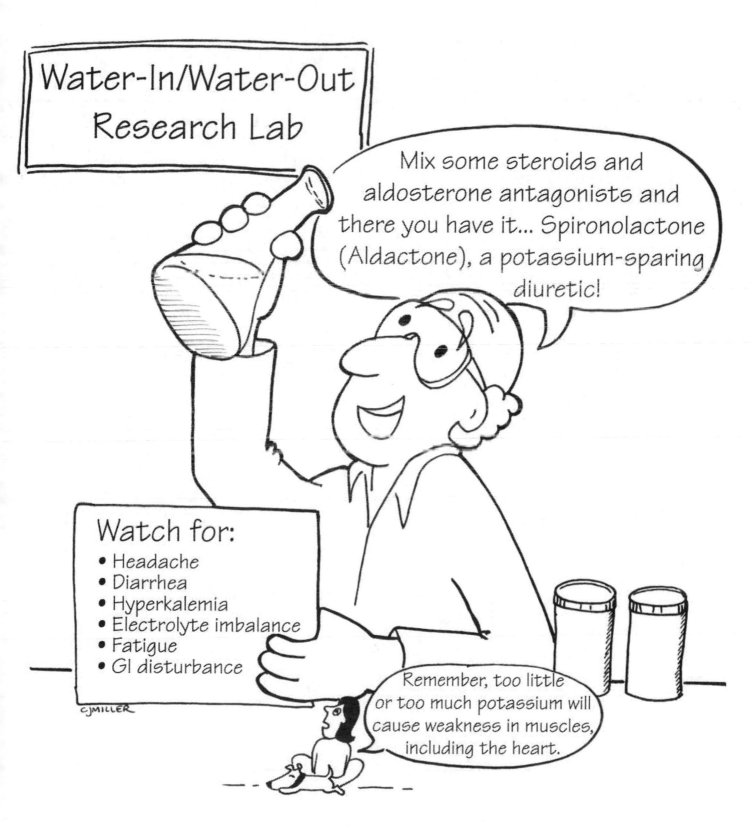

Memory Notebook of Nursing: Pharmacology & Diagnostics

Bumetanide (Bumex)

"Gets the Fluid on the Move"

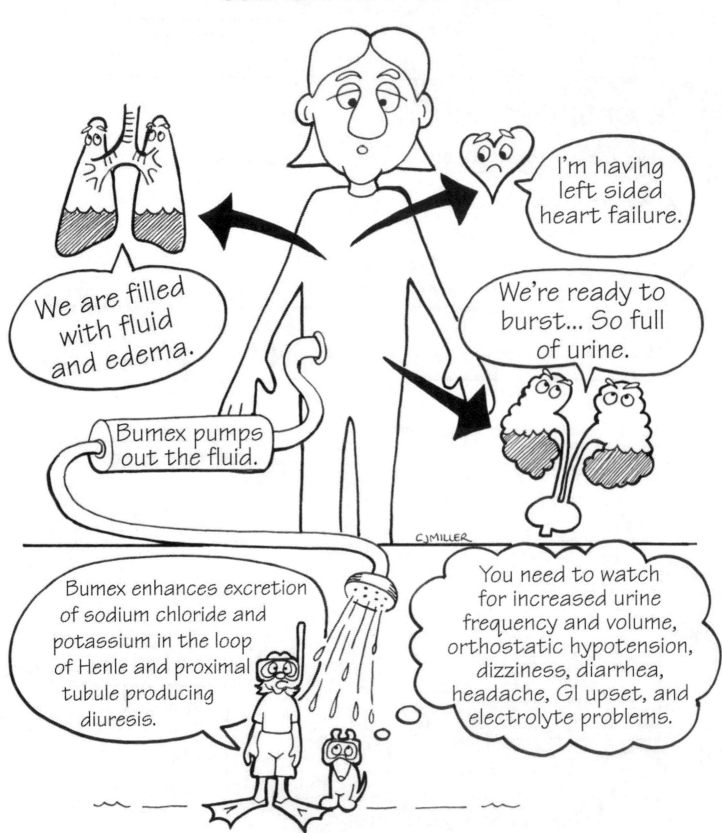

Diuretics
Memory Notebook of Nursing: Pharmacology & Diagnostics

The Diuretic Water Slide

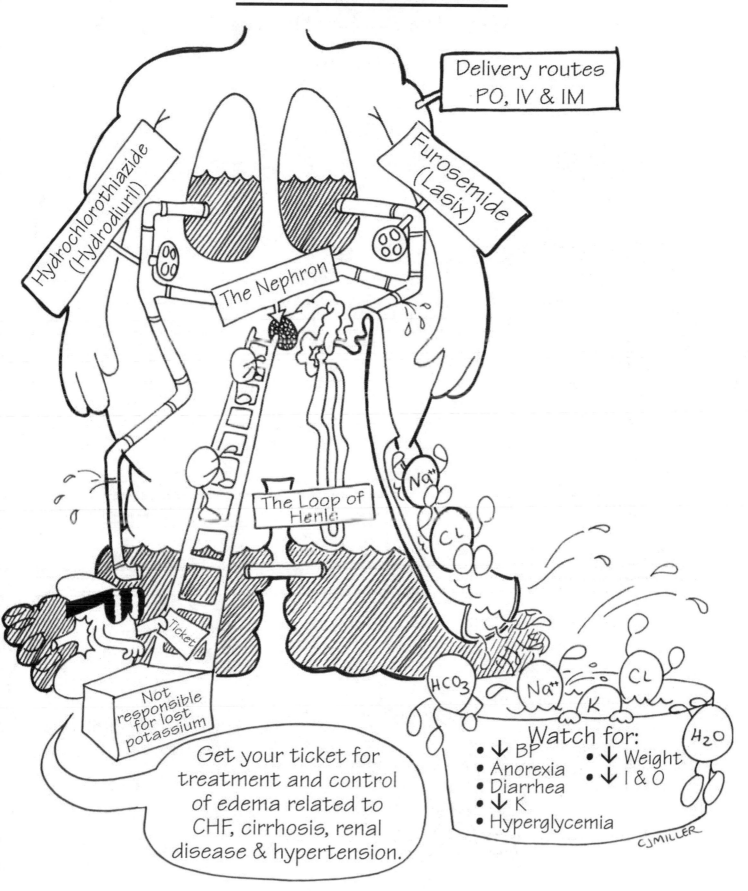

Delivery routes
PO, IV & IM

Hydrochlorothiazide
(Hydrodiuril)

Furosemide
(Lasix)

The Nephron

The Loop of Henle

Na⁺⁺

Cl

Ticket

Not responsible for lost potassium

Get your ticket for treatment and control of edema related to CHF, cirrhosis, renal disease & hypertension.

HCO3   Na⁺⁺   K   CL   H₂O

Watch for:
- ↓ BP
- Anorexia
- Diarrhea
- ↓ K
- Hyperglycemia
- ↓ Weight
- ↓ I & O

CJMILLER

Osmitrol
(Mannitol)

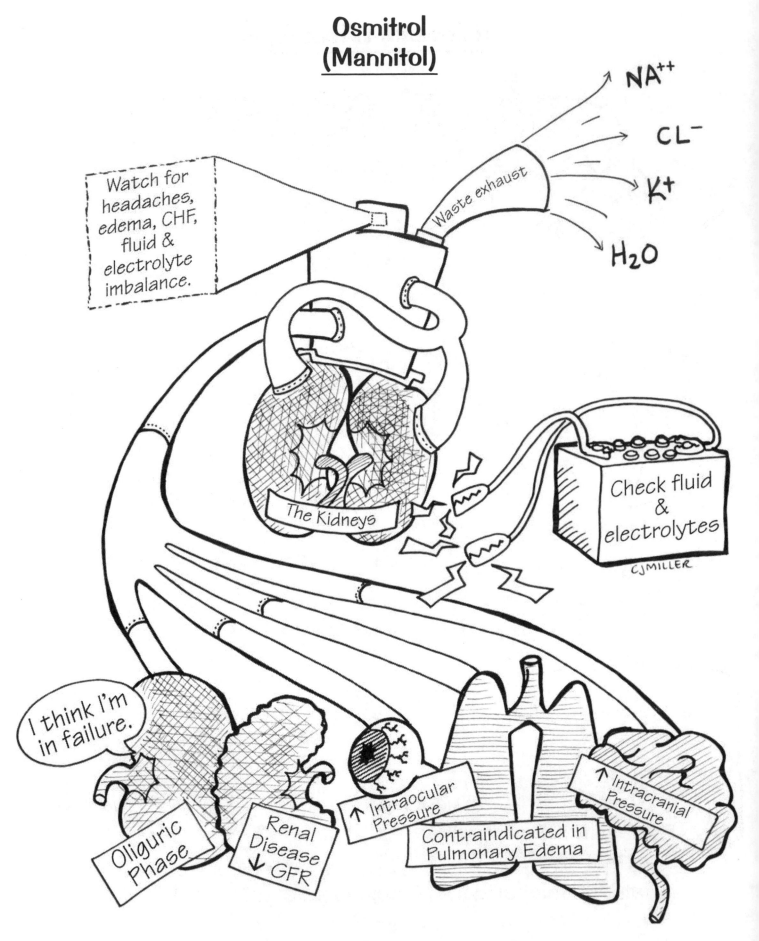

Haloperidol (Haldol)

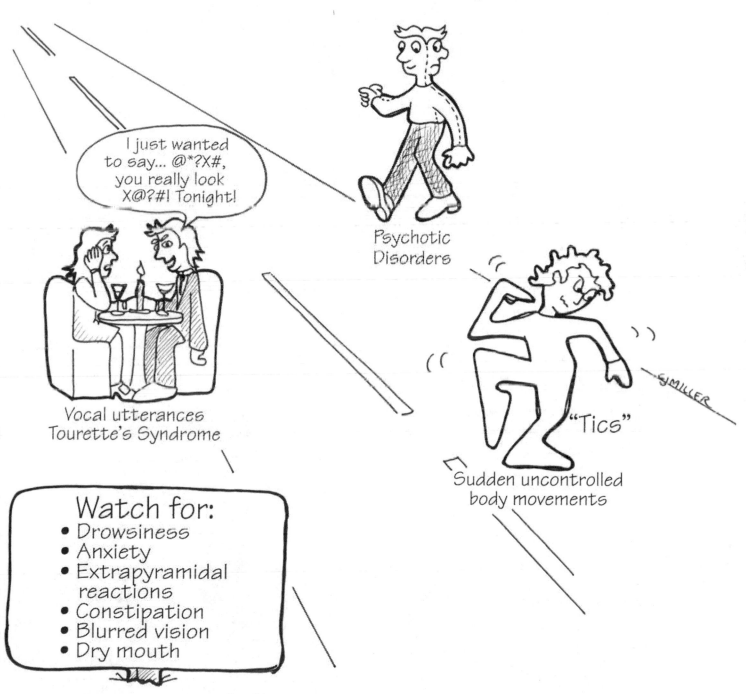

© 2005 Nursing Education Consultants, Inc.

MAO Inhibitors

Nardil, Marplan & Parnate

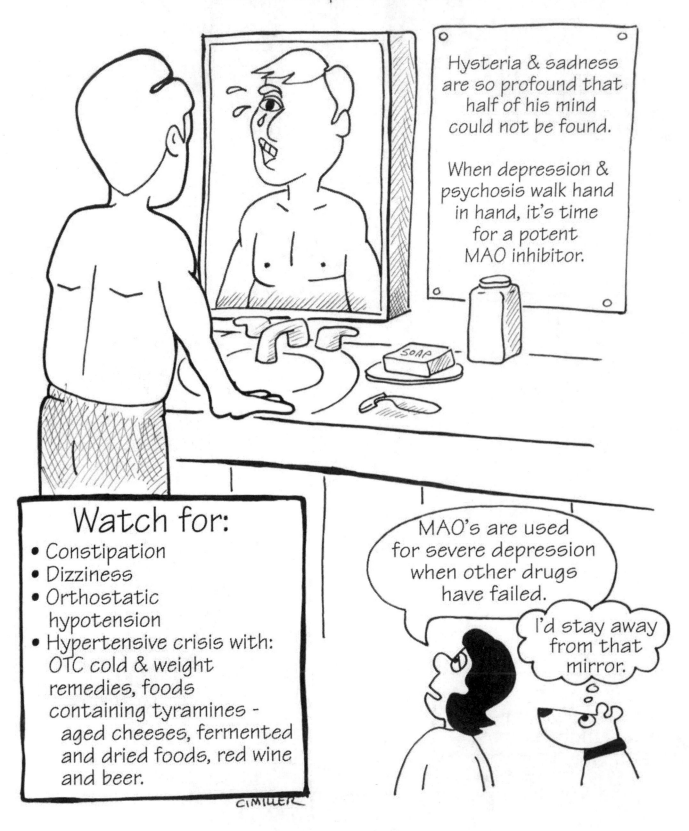

SSRI's

GET A GRIP ON LIFE
Dr. Feelgood's SSRI Traveling Show
Selective Serotonin-Reuptake Inhibitors

Stop obsessive thought and compulsive activities! Get rid of depression and anxiety!

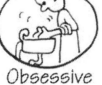
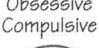
Obsessive Compulsive

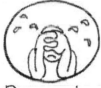
Depression

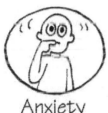
Anxiety

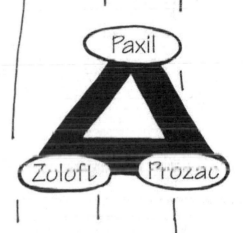
Paxil
Zoloft   Prozac

Watch for:
- Insomnia
- Palpitations
- Indigestion
- Diarrhea
- Sexual dysfunction

With Zoloft watch for delusions and aggressive behavior.

CJMILLER

Chlorpromazine (Thorazine)

"The Many Faces of Thorazine"

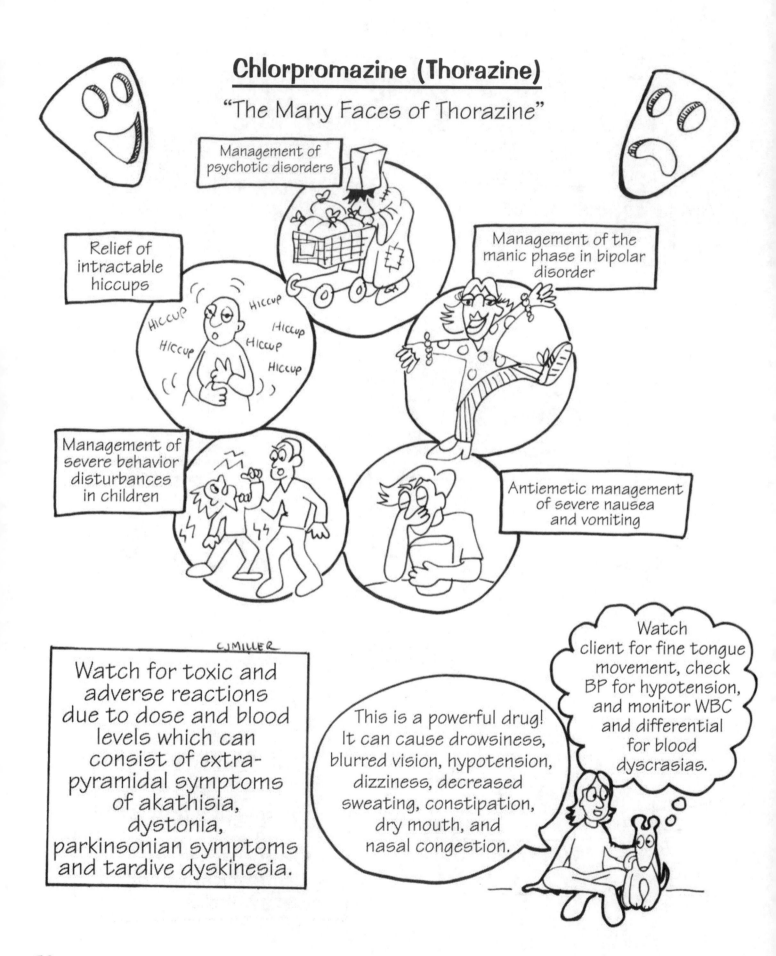

Management of psychotic disorders

Relief of intractable hiccups

Management of the manic phase in bipolar disorder

Management of severe behavior disturbances in children

Antiemetic management of severe nausea and vomiting

CJMILLER

Watch for toxic and adverse reactions due to dose and blood levels which can consist of extra-pyramidal symptoms of akathisia, dystonia, parkinsonian symptoms and tardive dyskinesia.

This is a powerful drug! It can cause drowsiness, blurred vision, hypotension, dizziness, decreased sweating, constipation, dry mouth, and nasal congestion.

Watch client for fine tongue movement, check BP for hypotension, and monitor WBC and differential for blood dyscrasias.

Tricyclic Antidepressants

 Amitriptyline
(Elavil)

 Doxepin
(Sinequan)

 Nortriptyline
(Pamelor)

 Imipramine
(Tofranil)

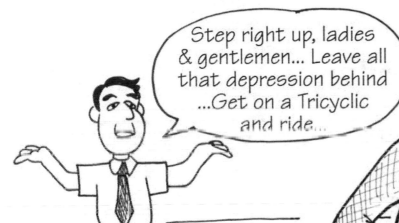

Step right up, ladies & gentlemen... Leave all that depression behind ...Get on a Tricyclic and ride...

I feel so much better on my Tricyclic.

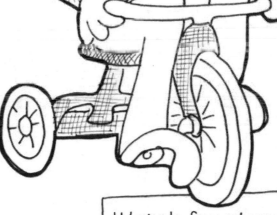

This classification is used for endogenous depression, reactive depression & depression related to alcohol & cocaine withdrawal.

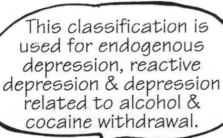
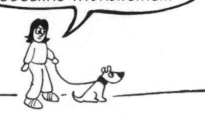

CJMILLER

Watch for signs of:
- Sedation
- Orthostatic Hypotension
- Headache
- Dry Mouth
- Urinary Retention
- Tachycardia

Bupropion (Wellbutrin and Zyban)

"Getting Well with Wellbutrin."

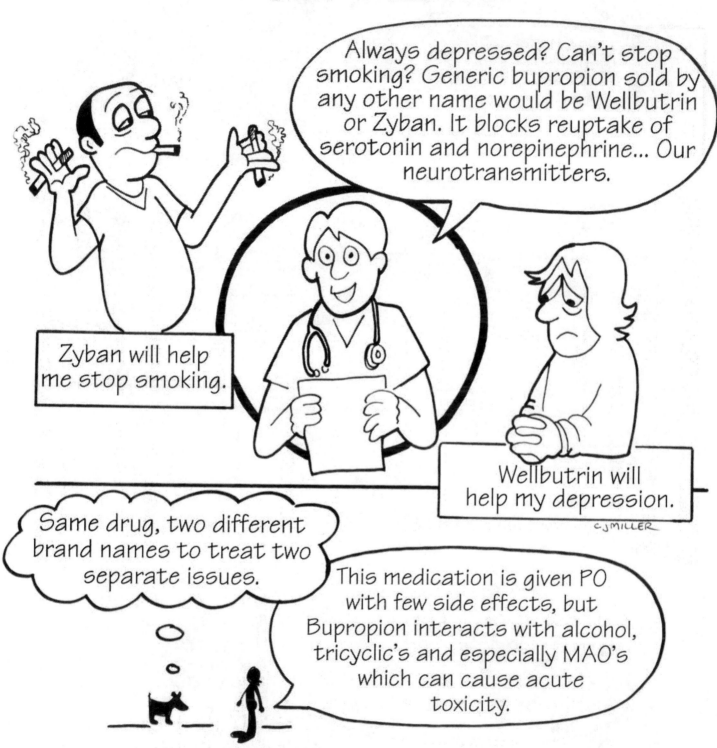

Glimepiride (Amaryl) and Glipizide (Glucotrol)

"Amaryl and Glucotrol - Releasing Insulin from the Beta Cells."

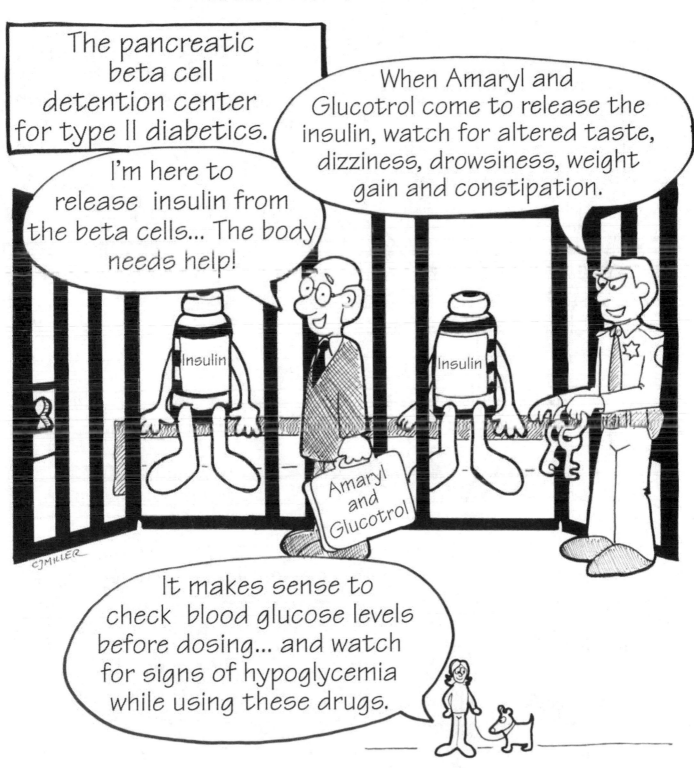

Calcitonin - salmon (Calcimar)

"When diet alone just isn't enough...
Calcimar, a bone resorption inhibitor."

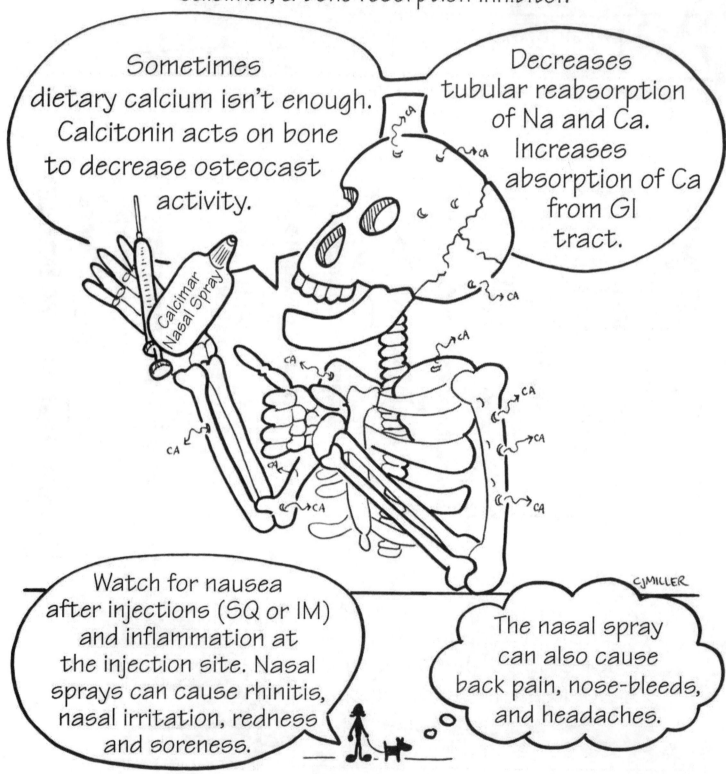

Endocrine
Memory Notebook of Nursing: Pharmacology & Diagnostics

Corticosteroids

Methylprednisolone (<u>Solu-Medrol</u>)
Dexamethasone (<u>Decadron</u>)
Prednisone (<u>Deltasone</u>)

Steroids... The Good, The Bad, and The Ugly!!!

These drugs stop, control or reduce the inflammatory response, (local or systemic) in any part of the body by suppressing the immune system.

The Good

Although there is a slow internal and external deterioration of the body, the trade off is that the steroid in a chronic or autoimmune disorder will usually keep the body alive longer than if the inflammatory process was left unchecked.

The Bad

The dose amount and duration of use dictate the extent of dependency and damage to the body. Watch for edema, peptic ulcers, delayed wound healing, osteoporosis & infections.

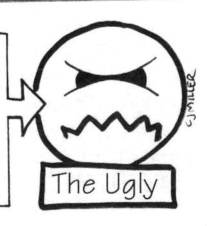

The Ugly

Glipizide (Glucotrol)

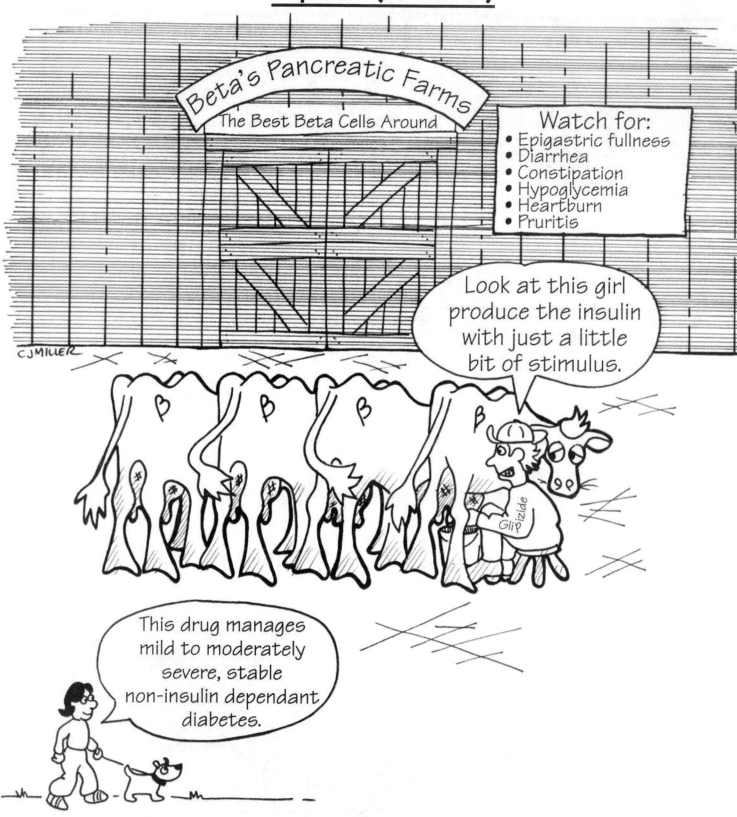

Endocrine
Memory Notebook of Nursing: Pharmacology & Diagnostics

Glucagon

"Glucagon, When the Sugar's Gone!"

A first aid kit for severe hypoglycemia

When the person is unable to remain conscious, glucagon is given SQ, IM or IV for emergency replacement.

Thanks for the brain candy... But watch for nausea, vomiting and hyperglycemia. The toxic effect can be hypokalemia.

This drug is reconstituted from a powder. Do not use unless solution is clear.

Brain candy, cool! The brain uses more glucose than any other body system.

Acarbose (Precose)

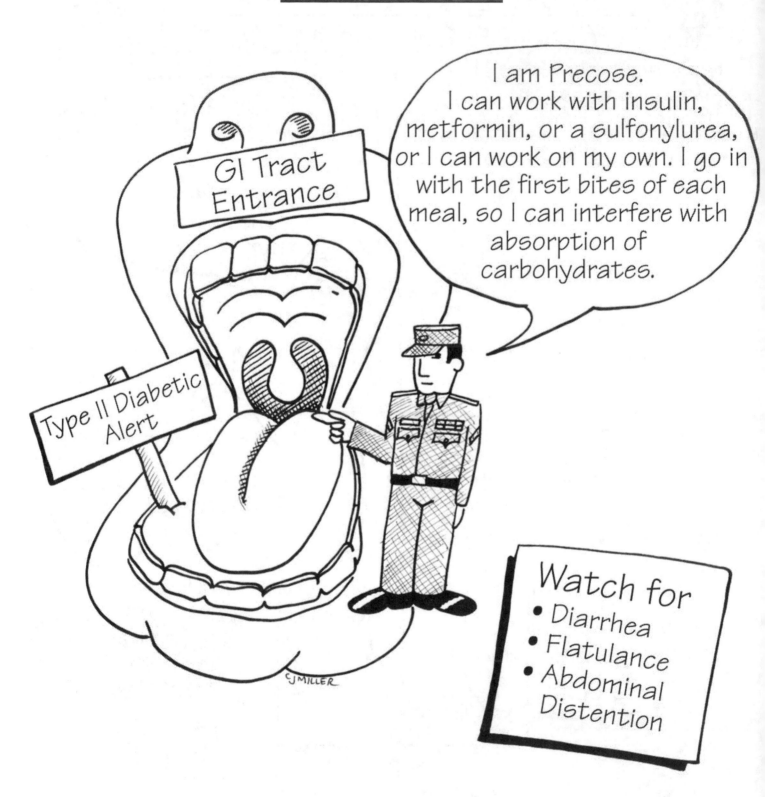

Rapid Acting Insulin

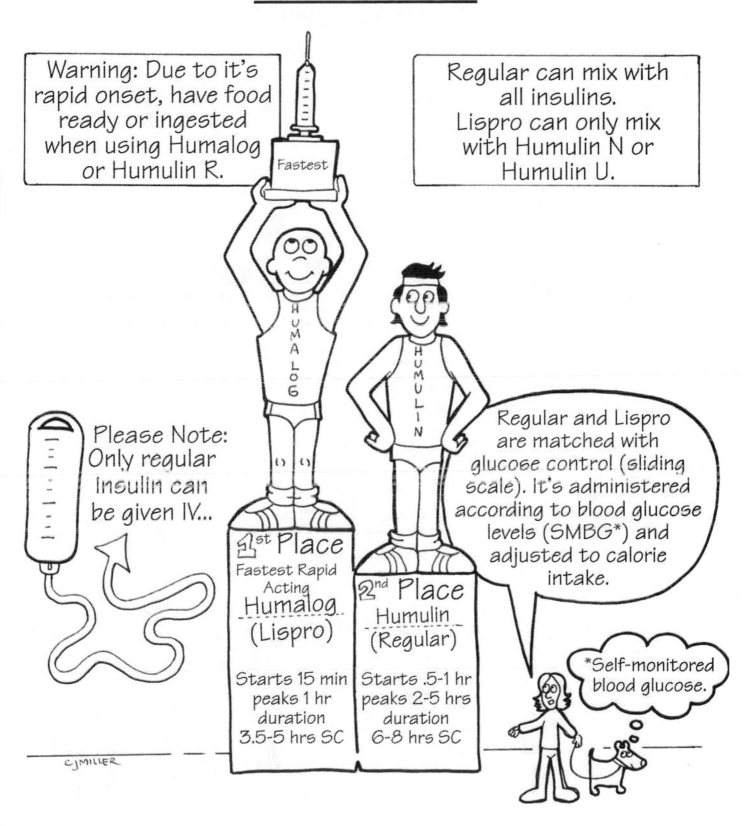

Warning: Due to it's rapid onset, have food ready or ingested when using Humalog or Humulin R.

Regular can mix with all insulins. Lispro can only mix with Humulin N or Humulin U.

Please Note: Only regular Insulin can be given IV...

Regular and Lispro are matched with glucose control (sliding scale). It's administered according to blood glucose levels (SMBG*) and adjusted to calorie intake.

*Self-monitored blood glucose.

Fastest

HUMALOG

HUMULIN

1st Place
Fastest Rapid Acting
Humalog
(Lispro)

Starts 15 min
peaks 1 hr
duration
3.5-5 hrs SC

2nd Place
Humulin
(Regular)

Starts .5-1 hr
peaks 2-5 hrs
duration
6-8 hrs SC

CJMILLER

Levothyroxine (Synthroid)

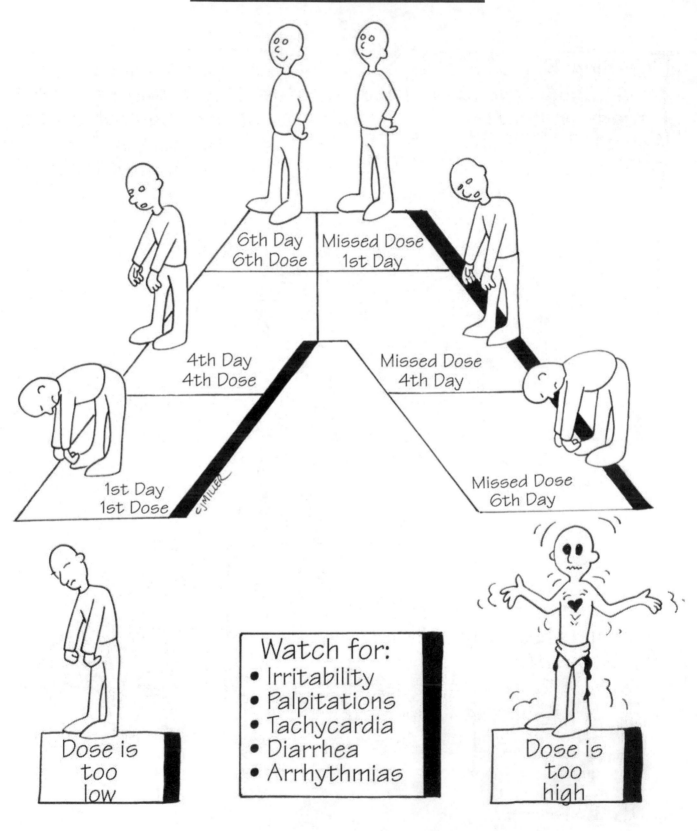

6th Day
6th Dose

Missed Dose
1st Day

4th Day
4th Dose

Missed Dose
4th Day

1st Day
1st Dose

Missed Dose
6th Day

Dose is
too
low

Watch for:
- Irritability
- Palpitations
- Tachycardia
- Diarrhea
- Arrhythmias

Dose is
too

Endocrine
Memory Notebook of Nursing: Pharmacology & Diagnostics

Methimazole (Tapazole)

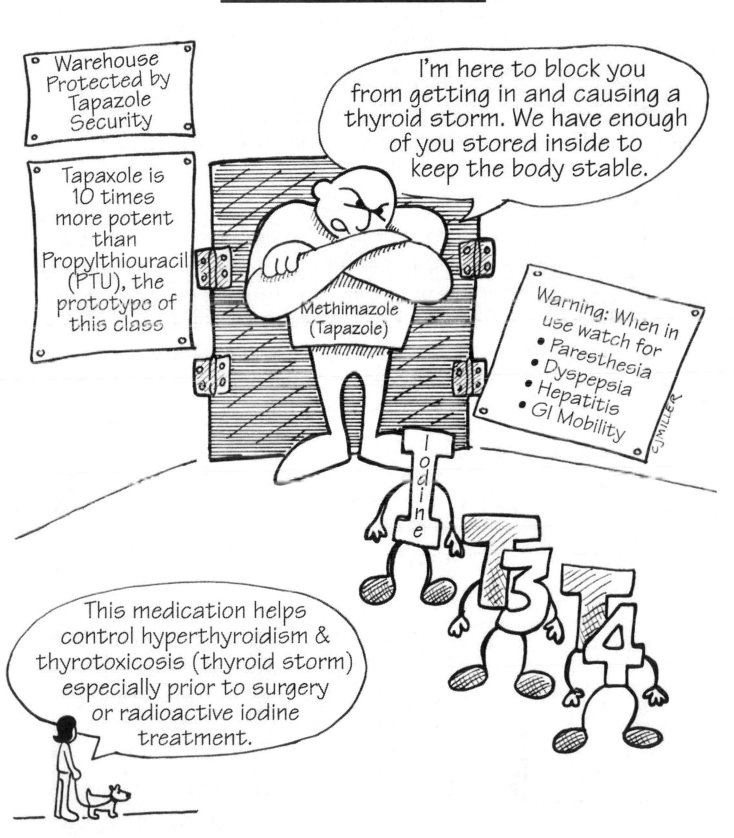

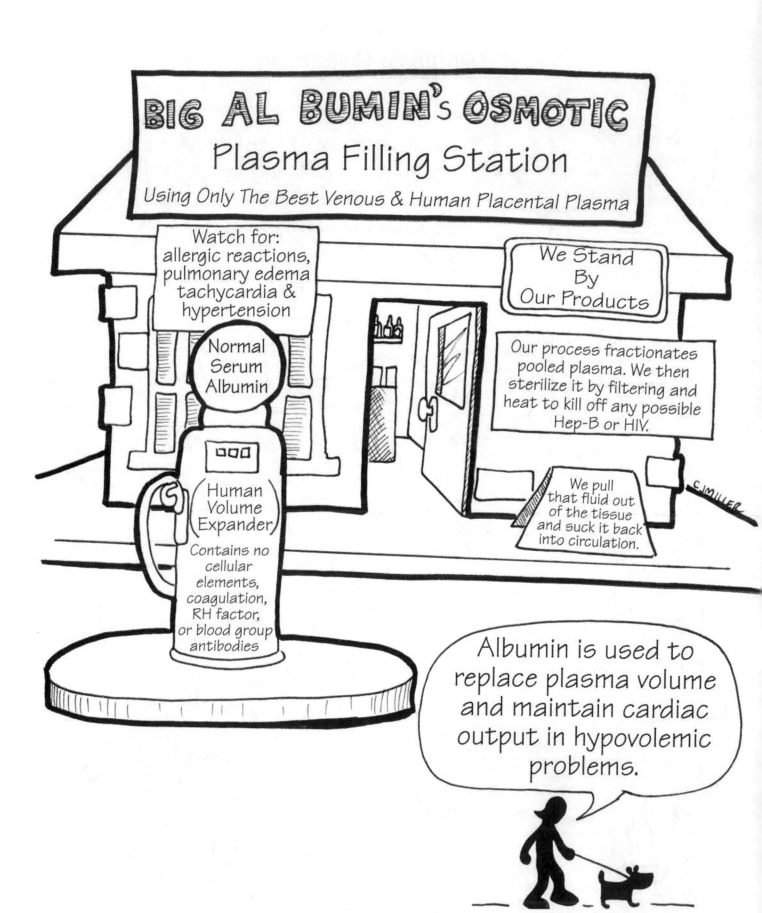

Endocrine
Memory Notebook of Nursing: Pharmacology & Diagnostics

Antifibrinolytics

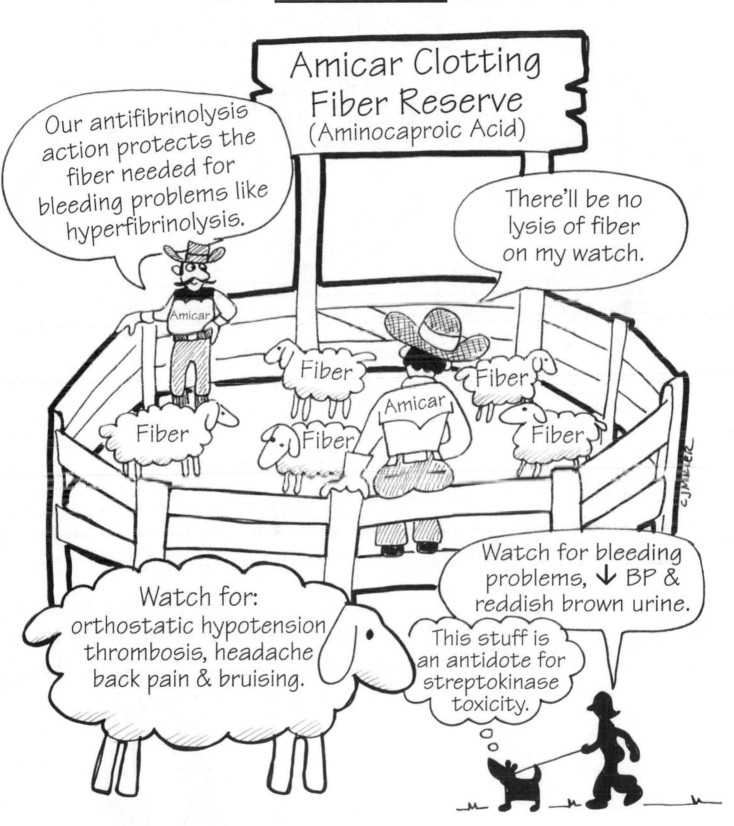

Warfarin Sodium (Coumadin)

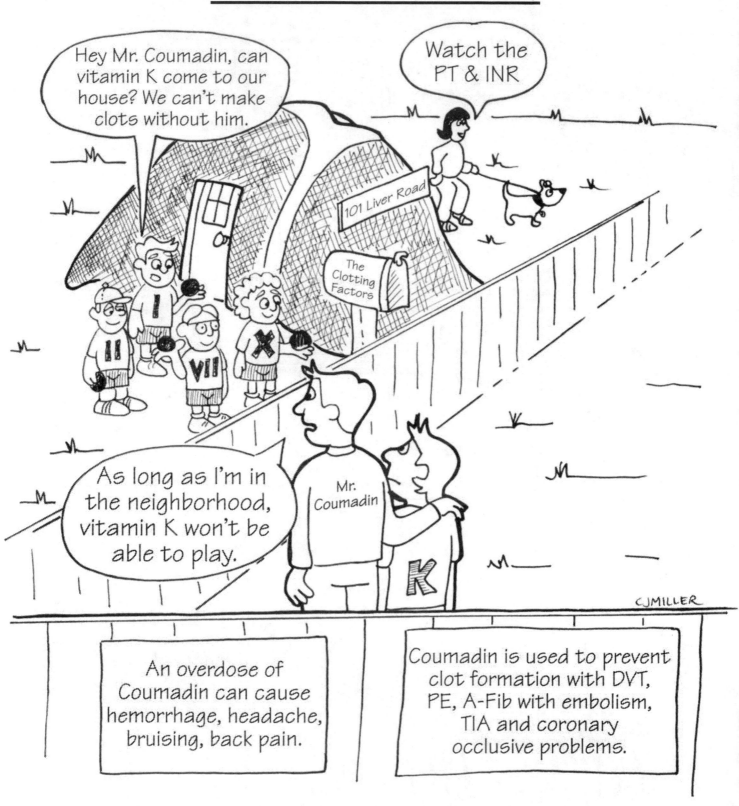

Heparin

"Controlling the Conversion Relay"

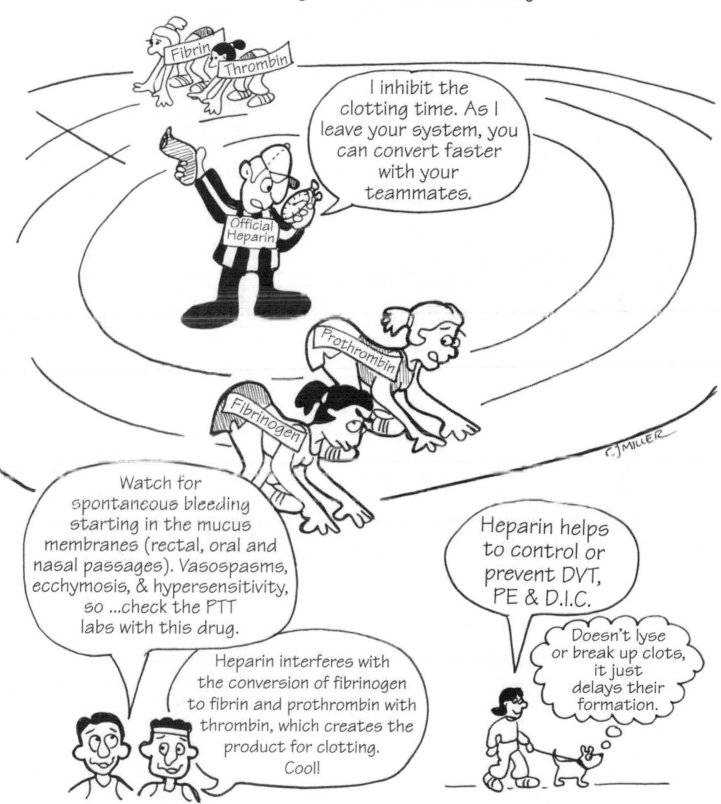

Iron Supplements

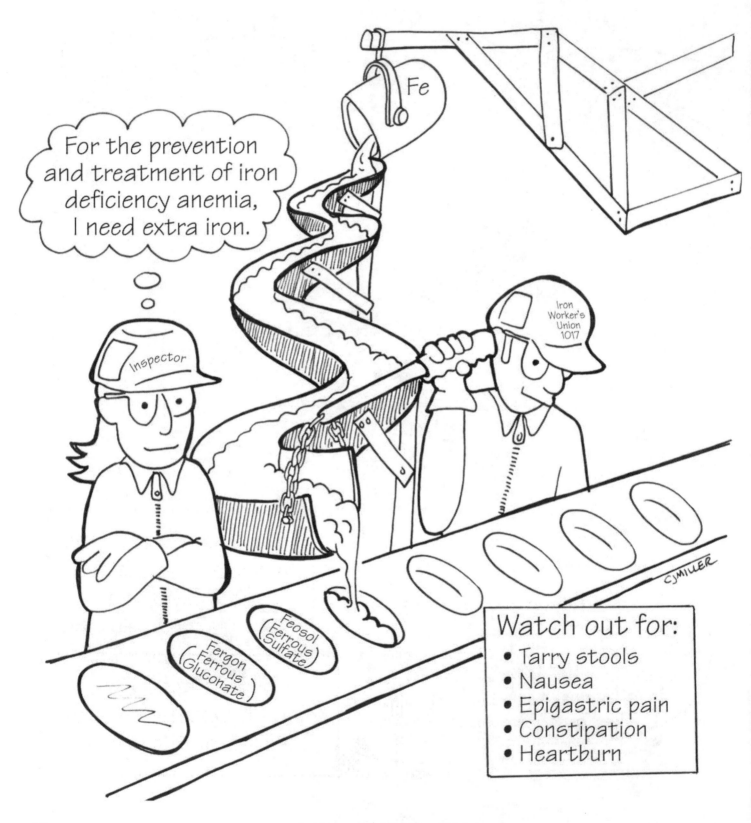

Cilostazol (Pletal)

"When Platelets Gather Together, Use Pletal for Crowd Control"

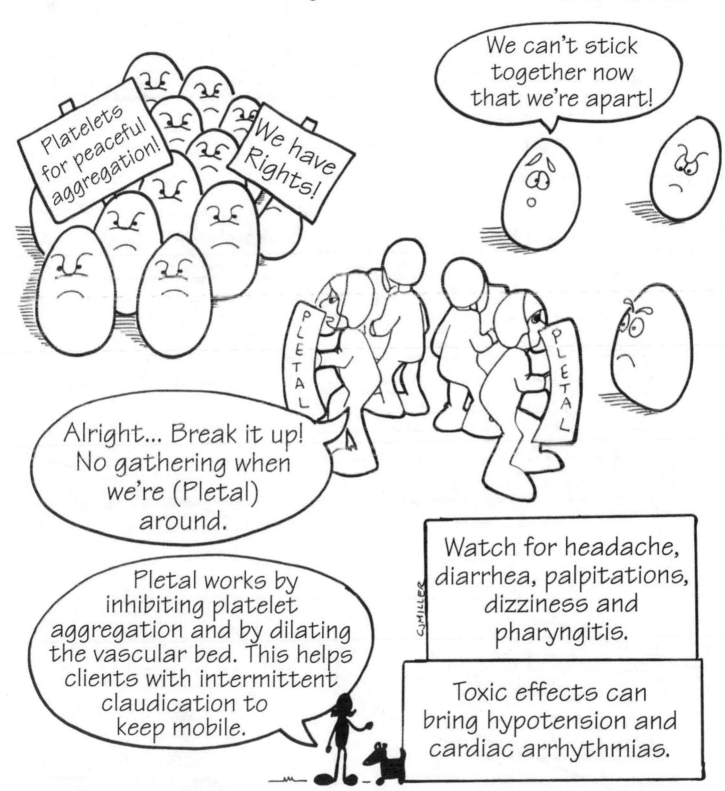

Epoetin Alfa (Procrit)

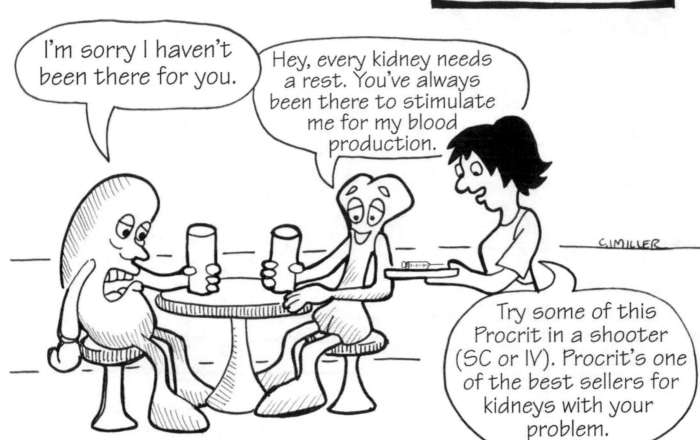

Procrit Juice Bar
Carrot Juice 8 oz $1.50
Celery Juice 8 oz $1.25
Procrit Market Price (SC/IV)

I'm sorry I haven't been there for you.

Hey, every kidney needs a rest. You've always been there to stimulate me for my blood production.

Try some of this Procrit in a shooter (SC or IV). Procrit's one of the best sellers for kidneys with your problem.

Procrit is synthetic erythropoietin, which increases HCT. Associated with anemia due to renal failure. Watch for: Seizures, diarrhea, iron deficiency and thrombocytosis.

Monitor the BP in conjunction with the HCT & CBC with diff. Oh, and watch those platelets!

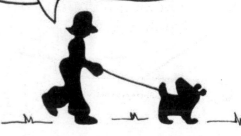

Anticoagulants / Hematinics
Memory Notebook of Nursing: Pharmacology & Diagnostics

Thrombolytics

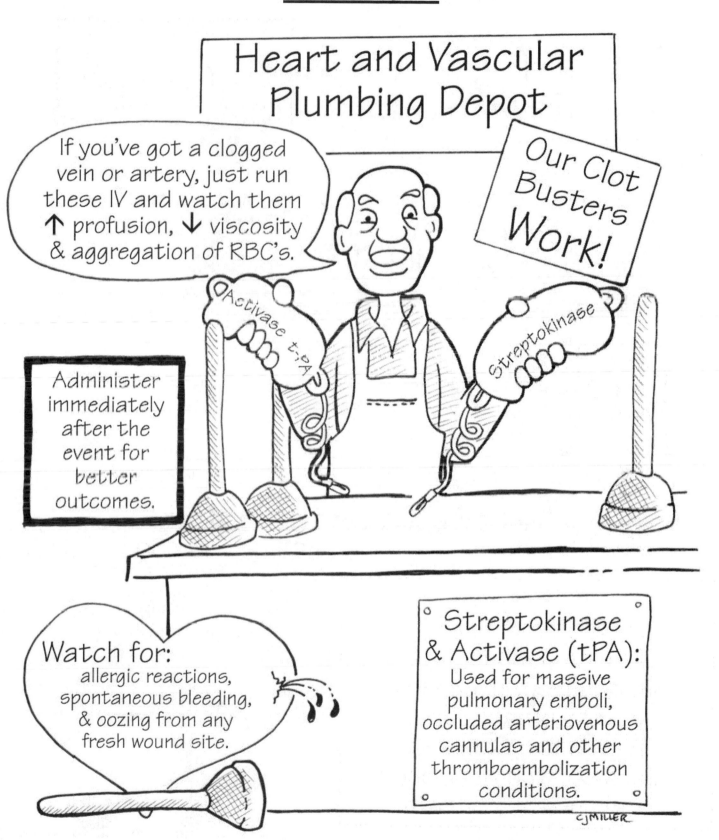

Aspirin

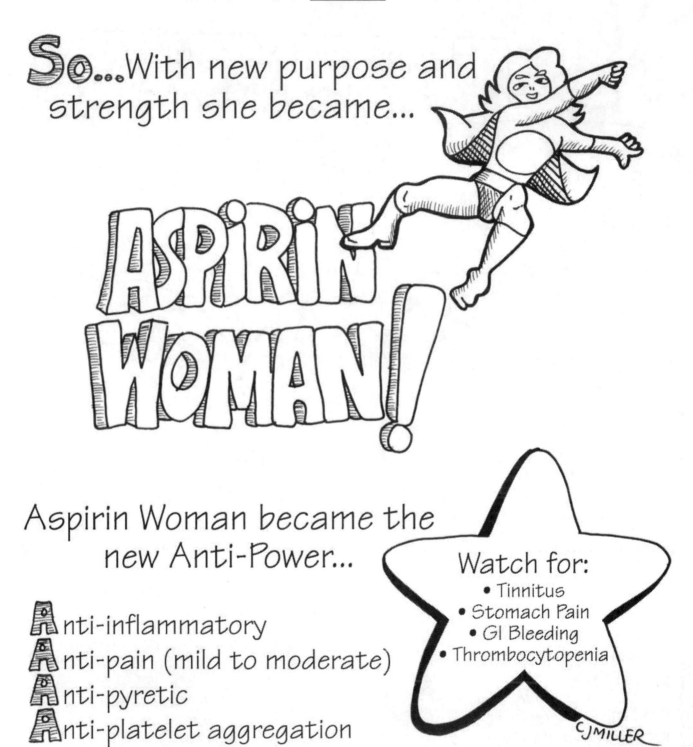

So...With new purpose and strength she became...

ASPIRIN WOMAN!

Aspirin Woman became the new Anti-Power...

Anti-inflammatory
Anti-pain (mild to moderate)
Anti-pyretic
Anti-platelet aggregation

Watch for:
- Tinnitus
- Stomach Pain
- GI Bleeding
- Thrombocytopenia

CJMILLER

Morphine Sulfate

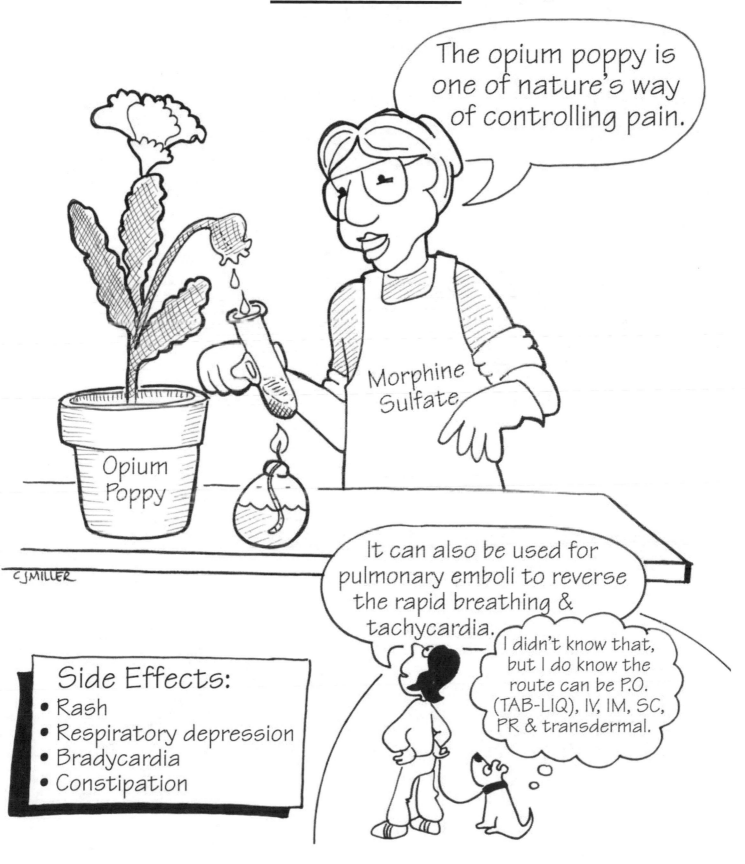

Memory Notebook of Nursing: Pharmacology & Diagnostics

Naloxone (Narcan)

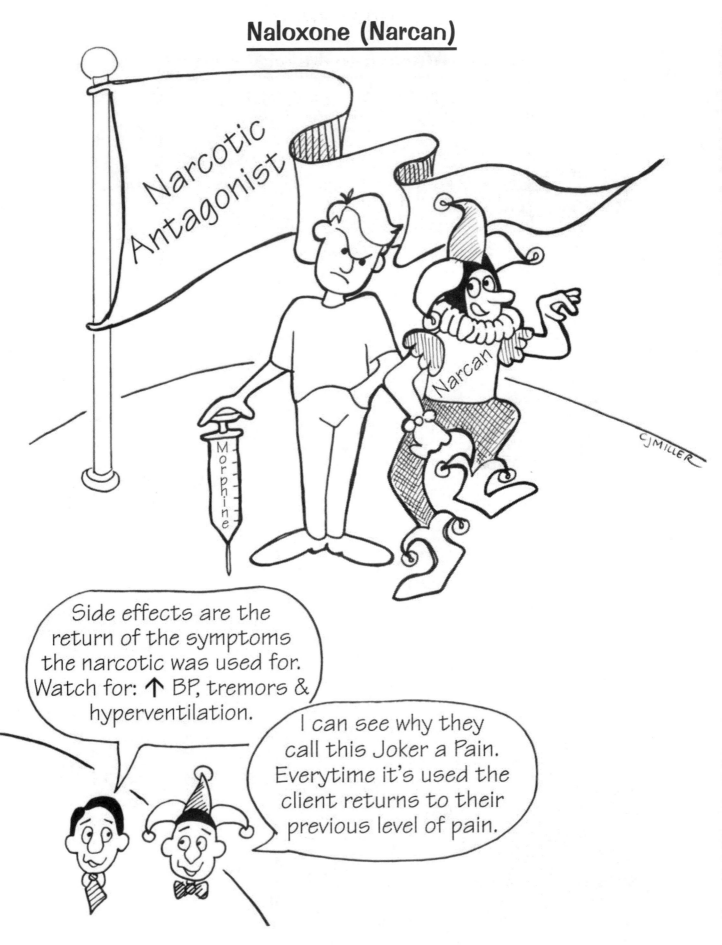

NSAID's

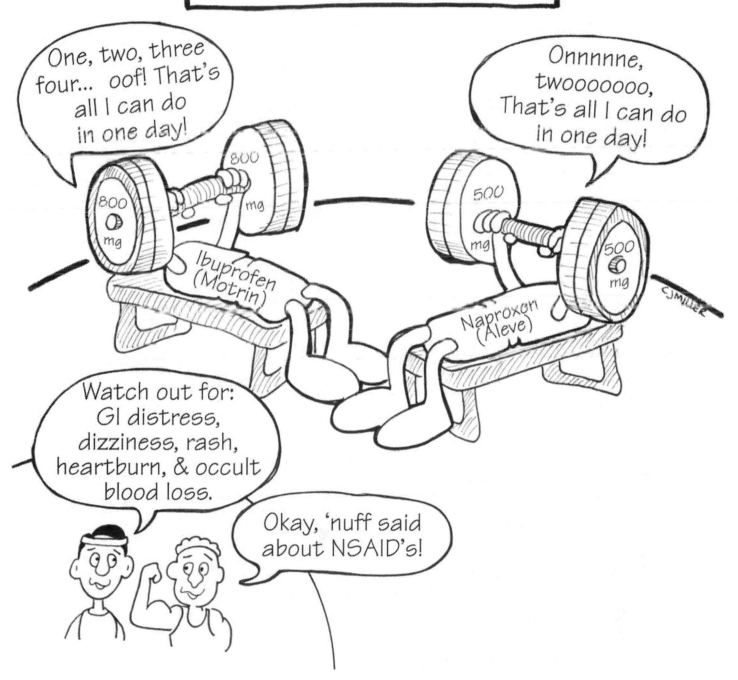

Antiseizure/Anticonvulsant

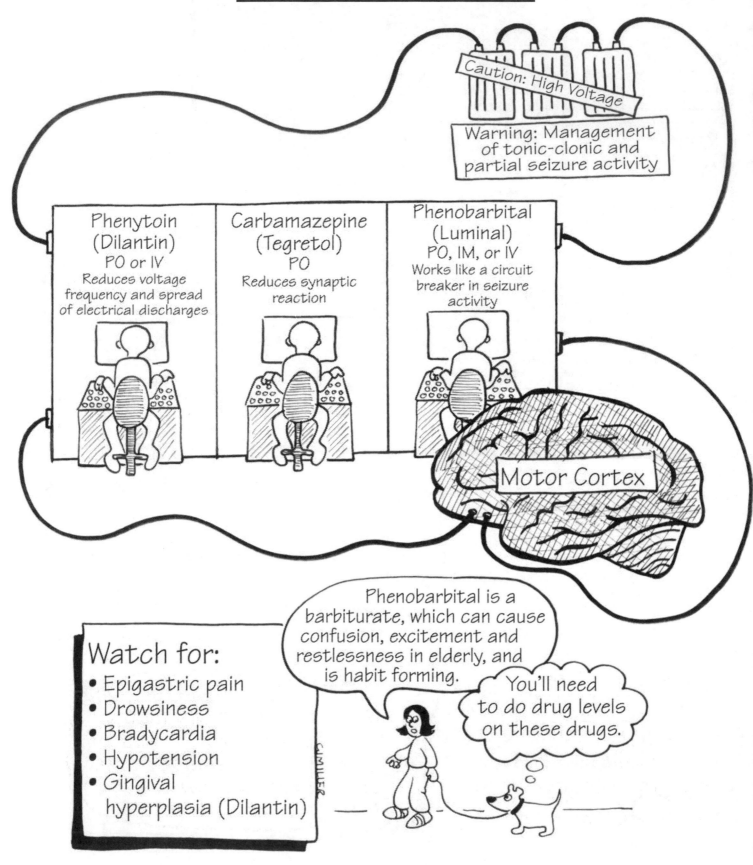

Neurologic and Sensory
Memory Notebook of Nursing: Pharmacology & Diagnostics

Benztropine (Cogentin)

"Controlling The Uncontrollable"
Anticholinergic; Antiparkinson Drug

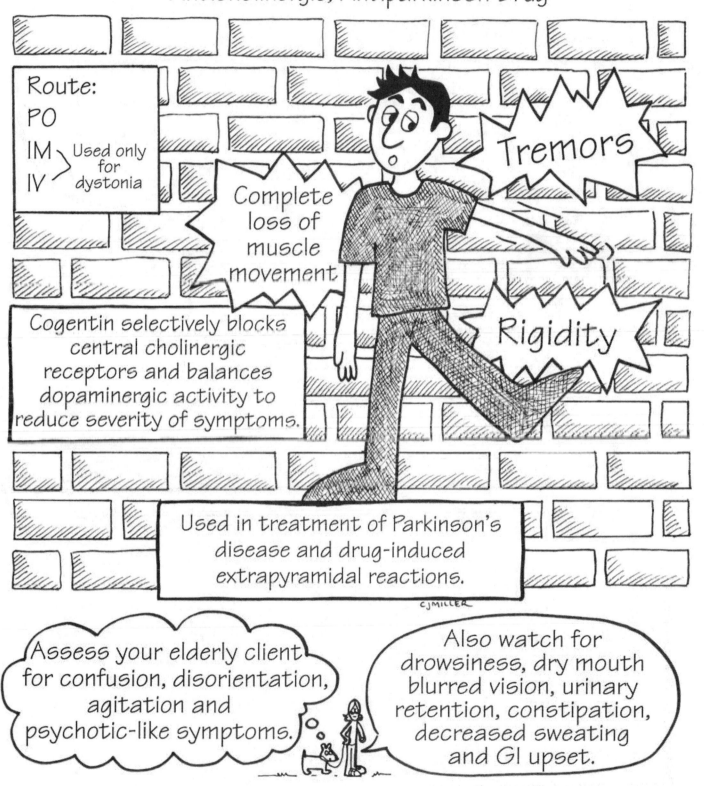

Route:
PO
IM } Used only for dystonia
IV

Complete loss of muscle movement

Tremors

Rigidity

Cogentin selectively blocks central cholinergic receptors and balances dopaminergic activity to reduce severity of symptoms.

Used in treatment of Parkinson's disease and drug-induced extrapyramidal reactions.

CJMILLER

Assess your elderly client for confusion, disorientation, agitation and psychotic-like symptoms.

Also watch for drowsiness, dry mouth blurred vision, urinary retention, constipation, decreased sweating and GI upset.

Clonazepam (Klonopin)

"Benzodiazepine and Anticonvulsant...
...Two sides to the Story."

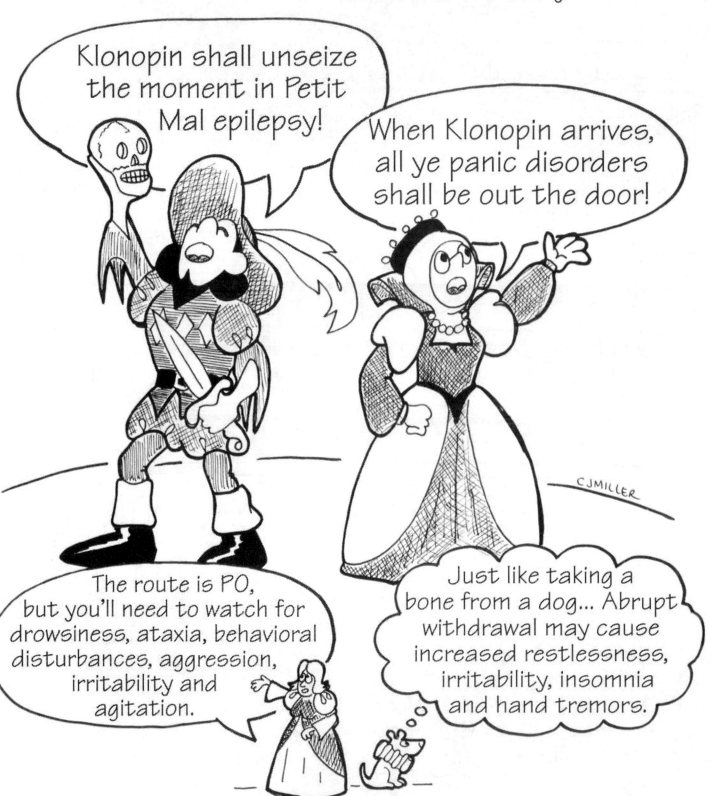

Neurologic and Sensory
Memory Notebook of Nursing: Pharmacology & Diagnostics

Gabapentin (Neurontin)

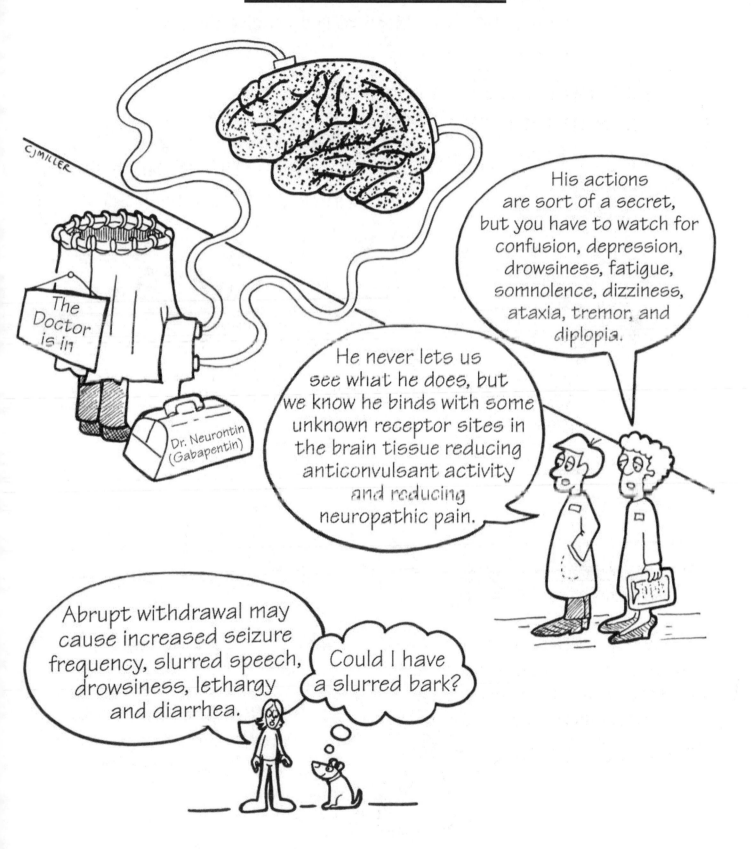

Carbamazepine (Tegretol)

"Stop the Seizures Before They Start"

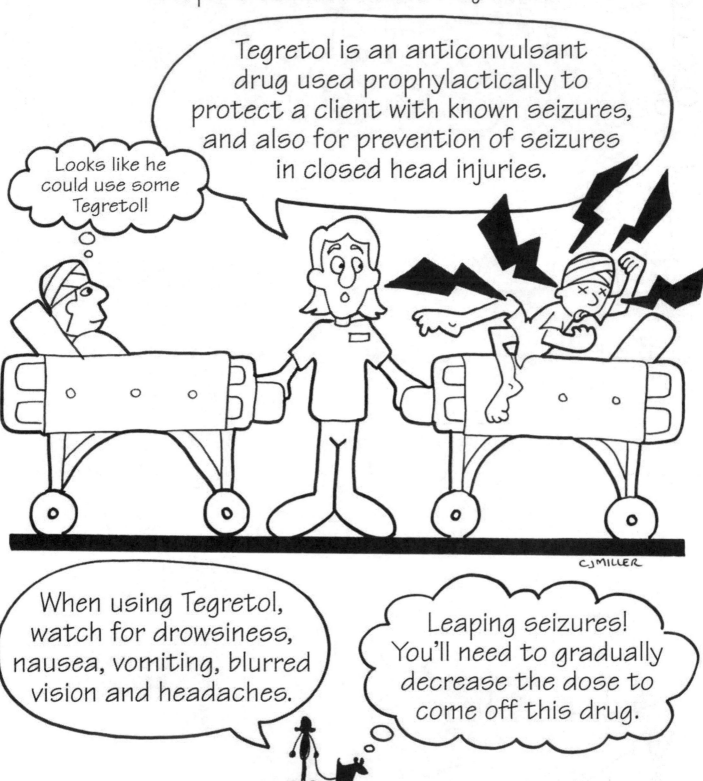

Neurologic and Sensory
Memory Notebook of Nursing: Pharmacology & Diagnostics

Timolol (Timoptic)

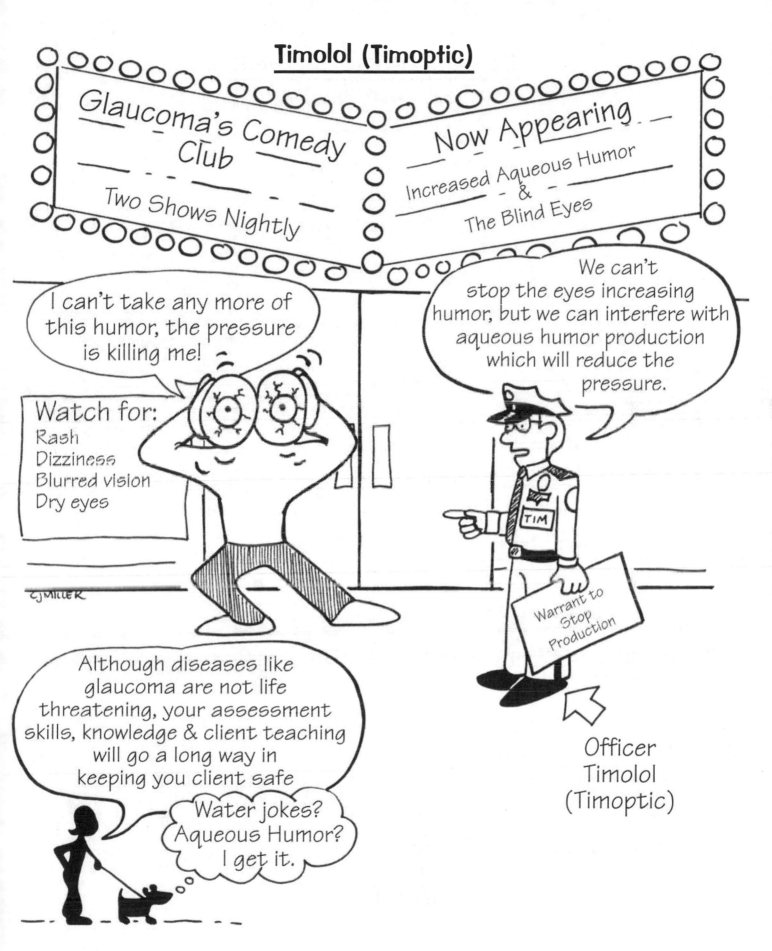

Topical Vasoconstrictor

Naphazoline (Clear Eyes) and Pseudoephedrine (Afrin)

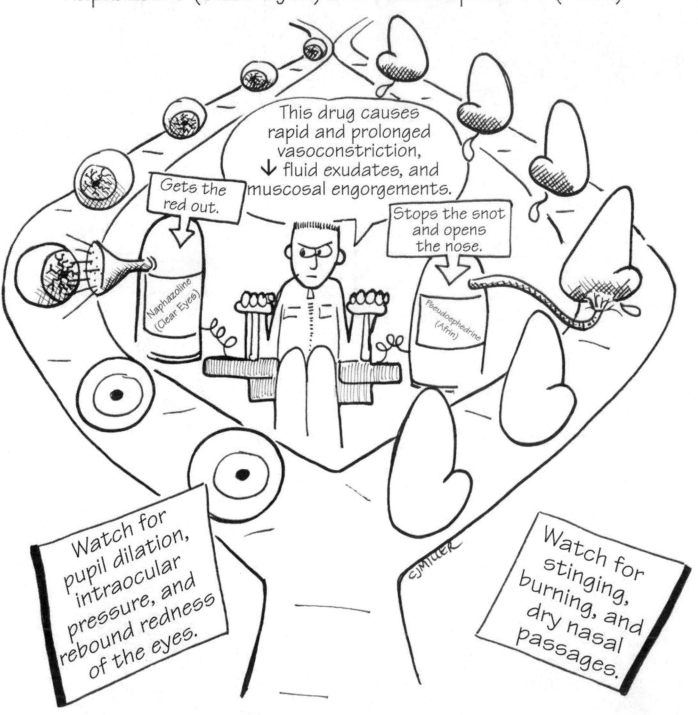

Antigout

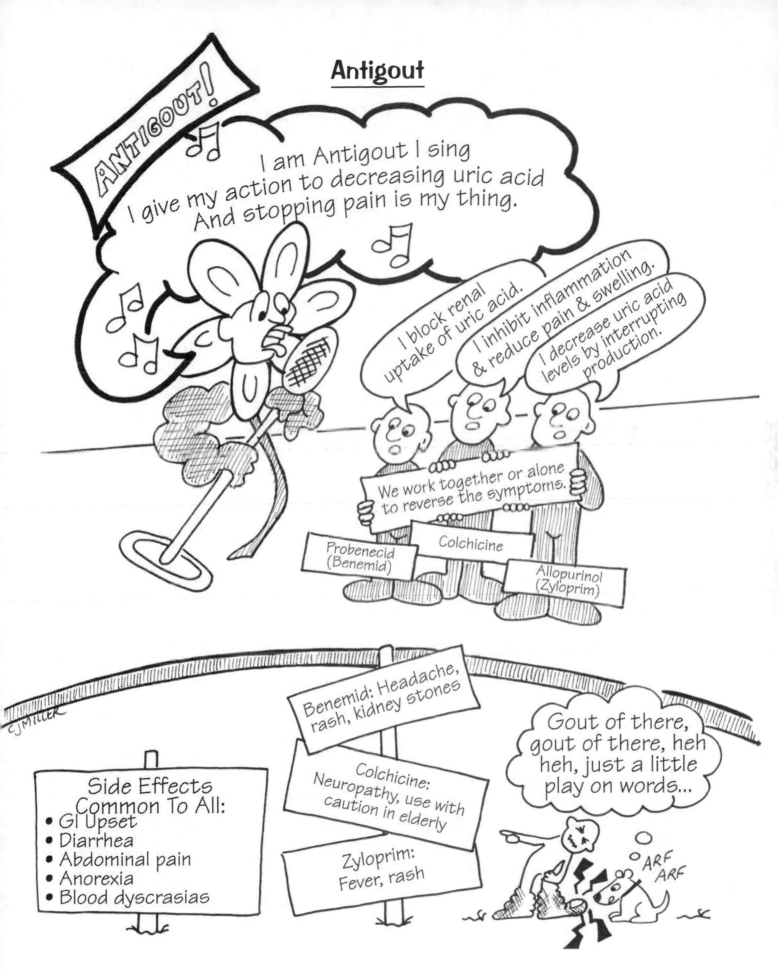

Colecoxib (Celebrex)

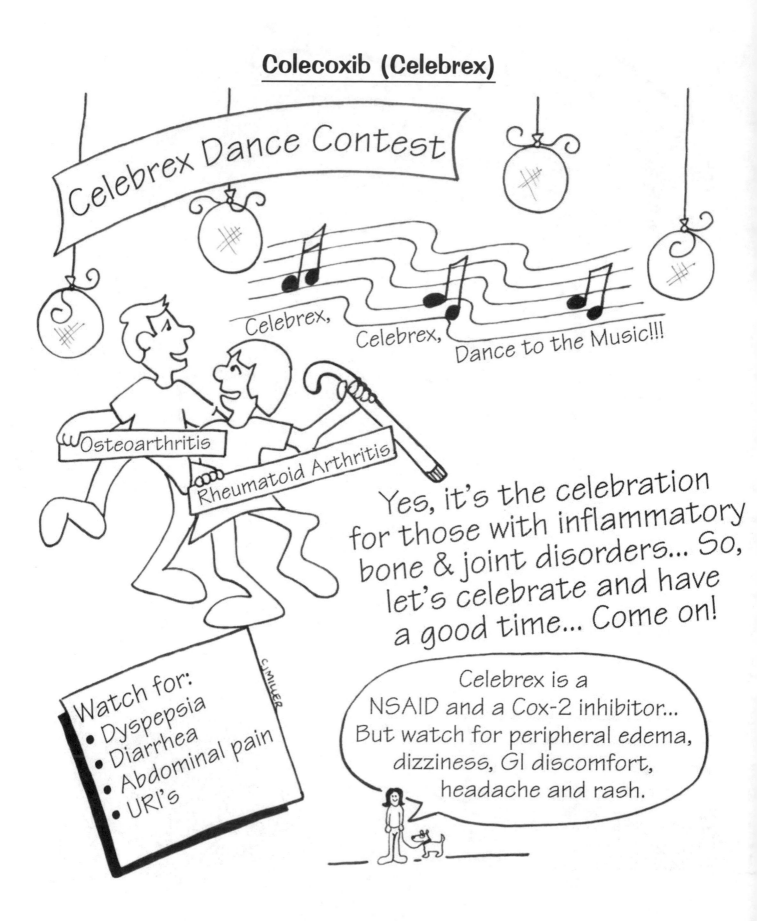

Alendronate (Fosamax)

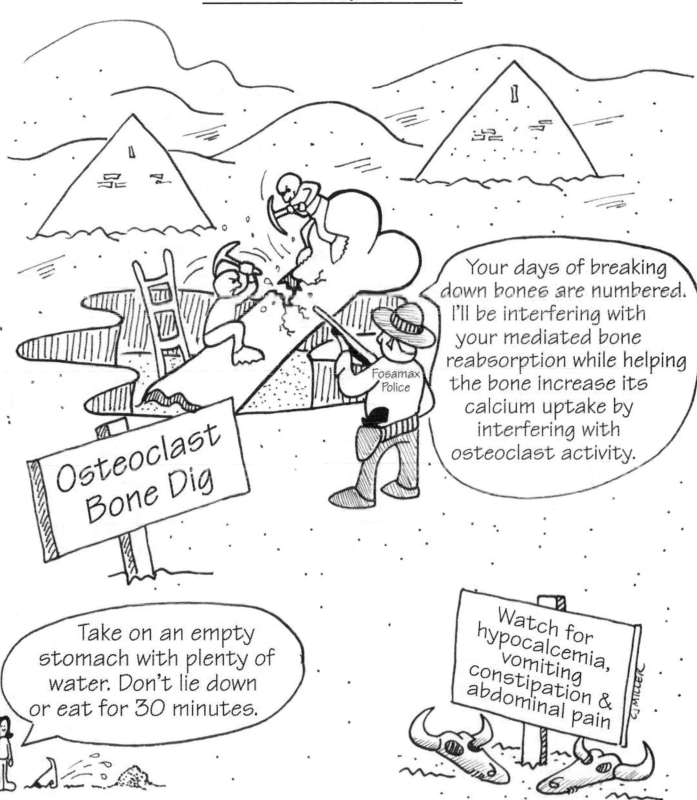

Etodolac (Lodine)

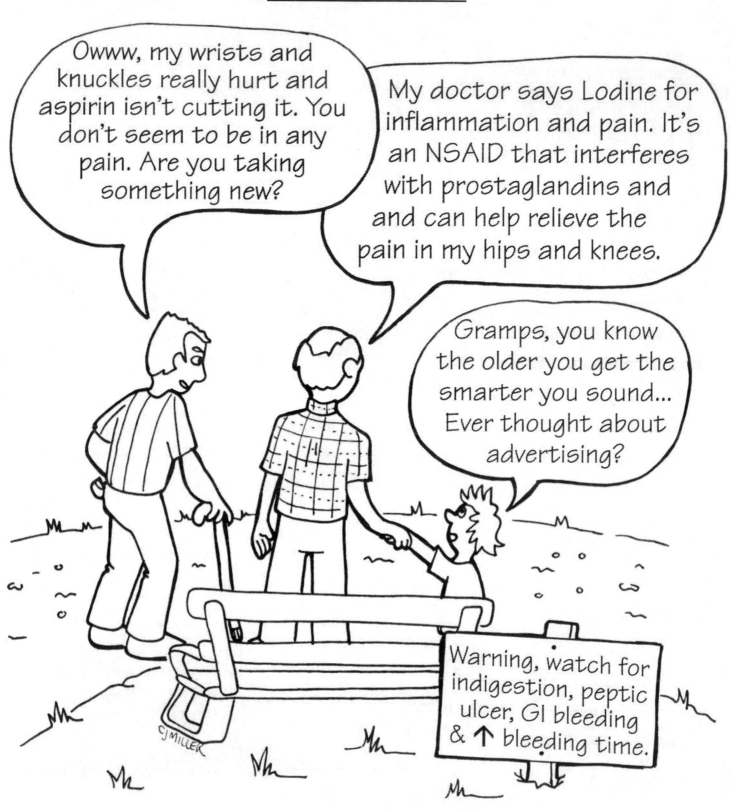

Medroxyprogesterone (Depo-Provera)

"It's Not Just For Birth Control"

Depo-Provera
For treatment of:

- Endometrial hyperplasia
- Secondary amenorrhea
- Abnormal uterine bleeding
- Adjunct and pallative treatment of endometrial and renal carcinoma
- Pregnancy prevention

Depo-Provera inhibits secretion of pituitary gonadotropins in order to prevent maturation and ovulation, relax uterine and smooth muscles... And to restore hormonal balance.

CJMILLER

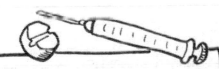

Can be administered IM (in the upper arm or outer aspect of the buttock) for contraception, one injection every 3 months.

You'll need to watch for transient menstrual abnormalities with initial use. Also watch for edema, weight change, breast tenderness, nervousness, fatigue and depression.

...Supresses ovulation, thickens cervical mucus and initiates secretory stage in the endometrium ...I have no idea where that came from.

Tolterodine (Detrol)

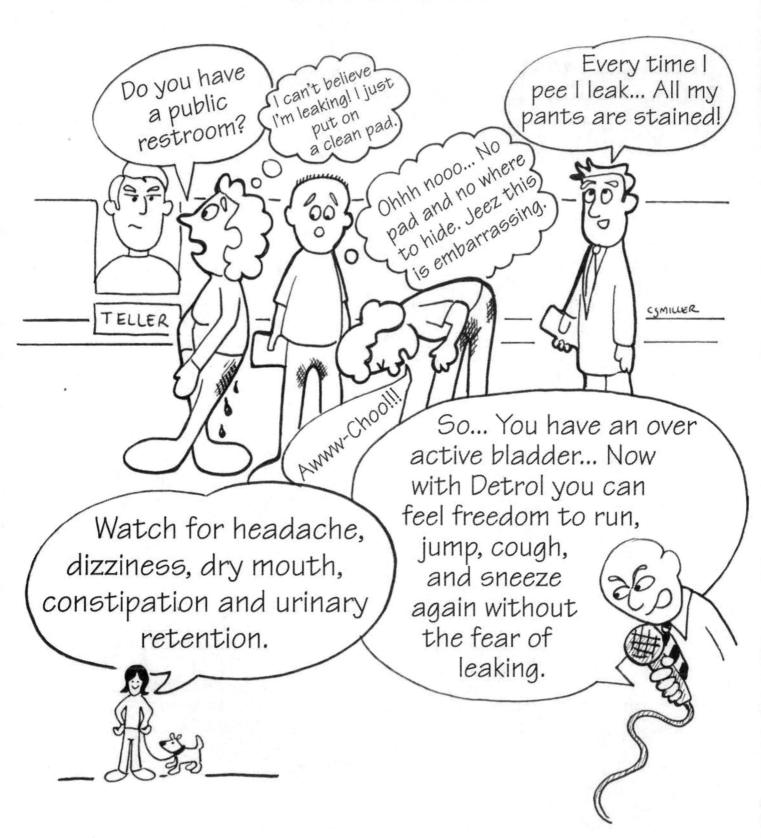

Hormone Replacement Therapy (Estrogen)

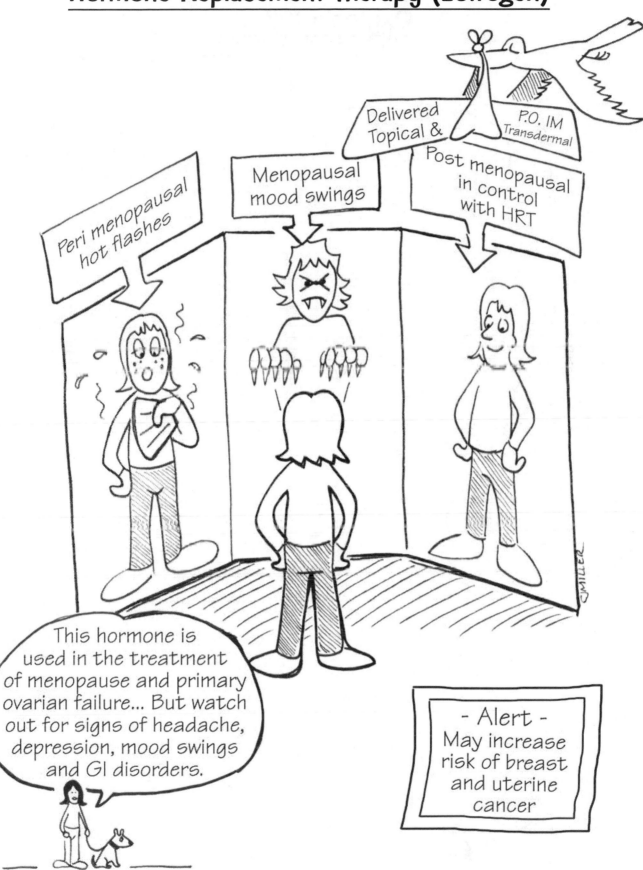

Oxytocin (Pitocin)

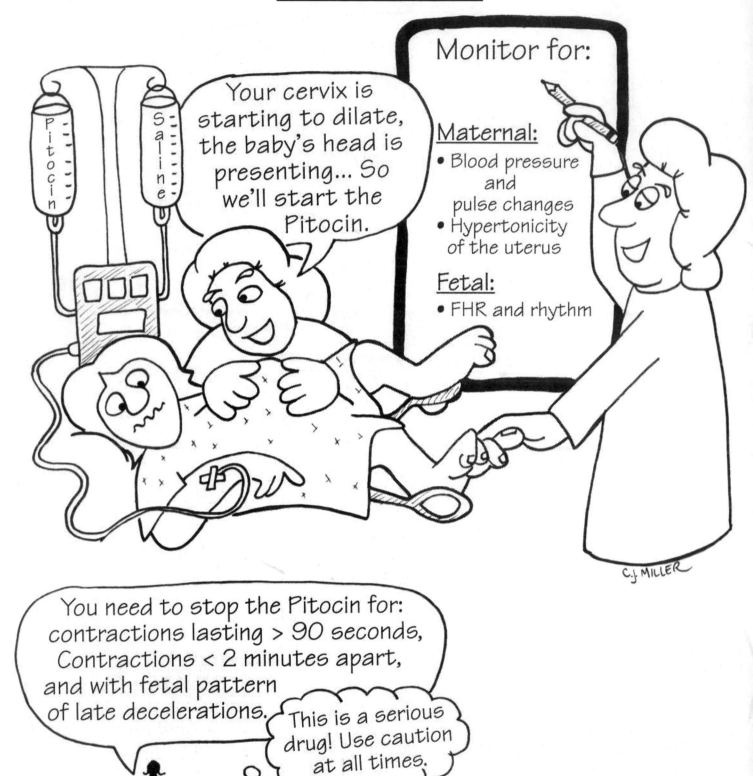

OB-Gyn
Memory Notebook of Nursing: Pharmacology & Diagnostics

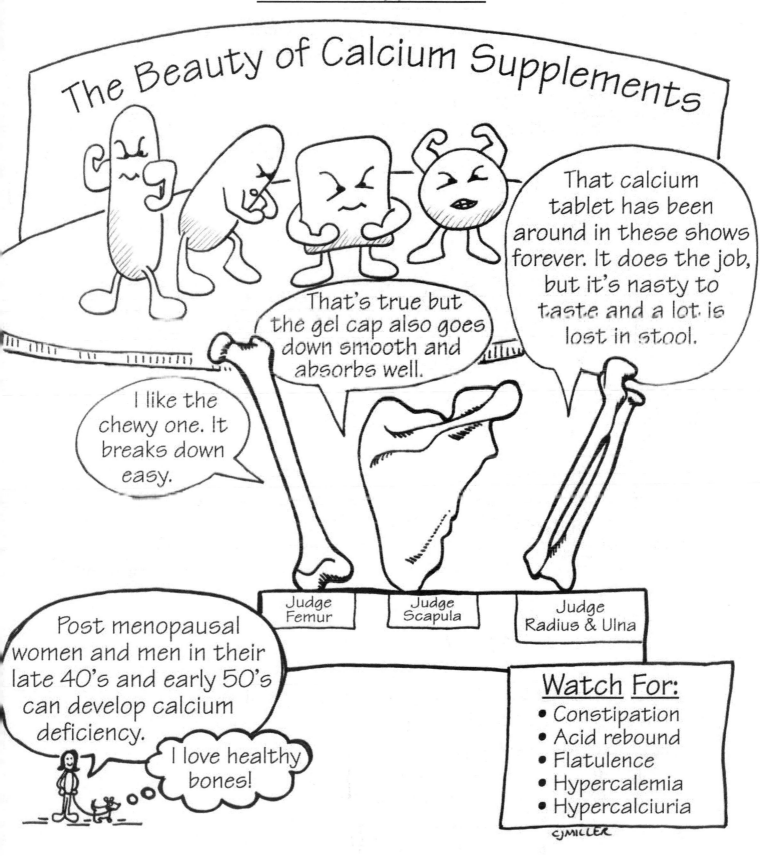

Calcium Supplements

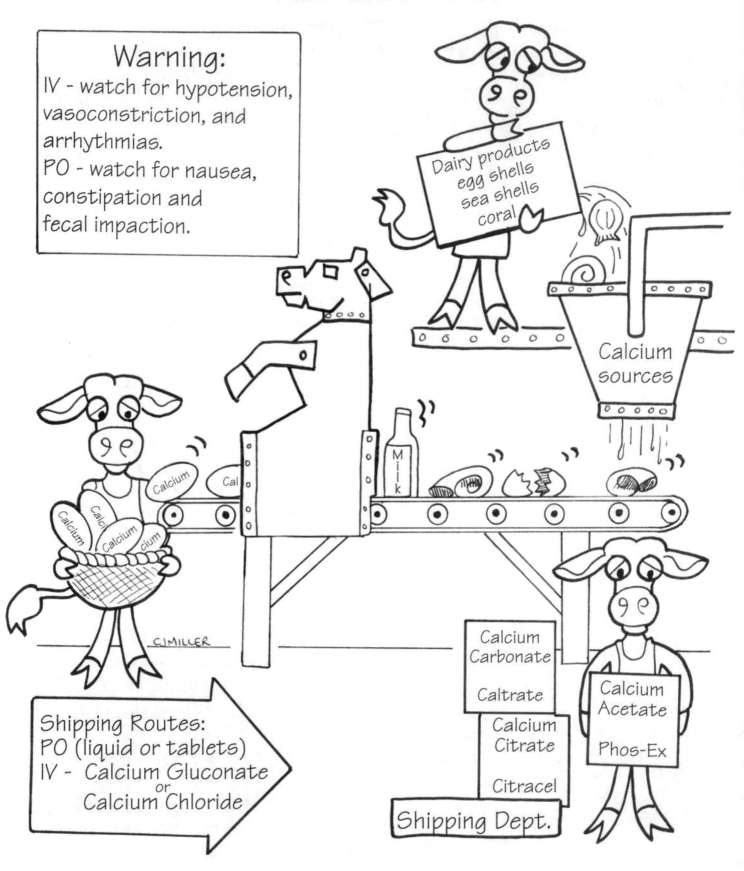

Warning:
IV - watch for hypotension, vasoconstriction, and arrhythmias.
PO - watch for nausea, constipation and fecal impaction.

Dairy products
egg shells
sea shells
coral

Calcium sources

Calcium

Milk

Calcium Carbonate
Caltrate
Calcium Citrate
Citracel

Shipping Dept.

Calcium Acetate
Phos-Ex

Shipping Routes:
PO (liquid or tablets)
IV - Calcium Gluconate
or
Calcium Chloride

CJMILLER

Miscellaneous
Memory Notebook of Nursing: Pharmacology & Diagnostics

Azathioprine (Imuran)

"Suppressing the Body's Defenses"

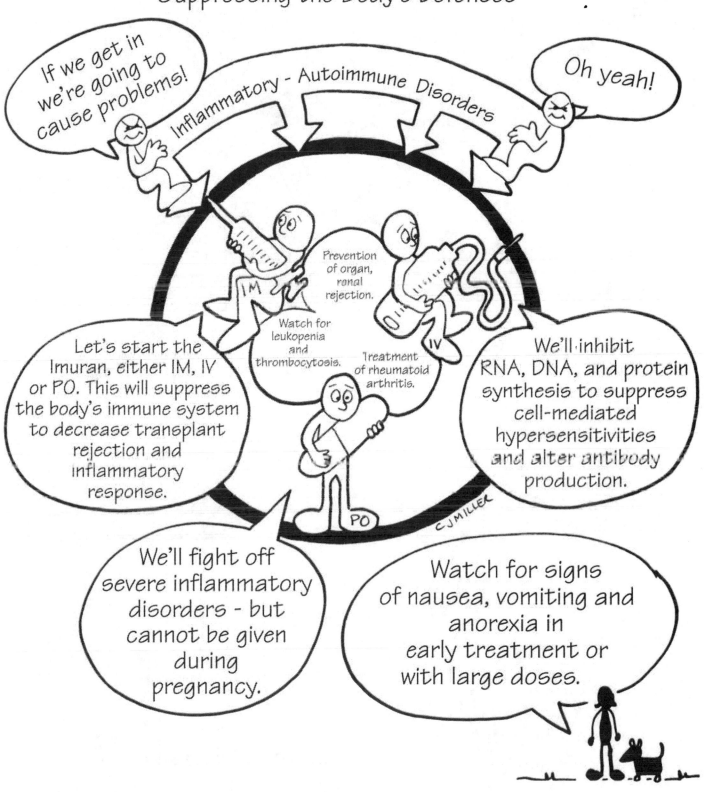

Potassium Chloride (K-Dur)

Life Hangs in the Balance

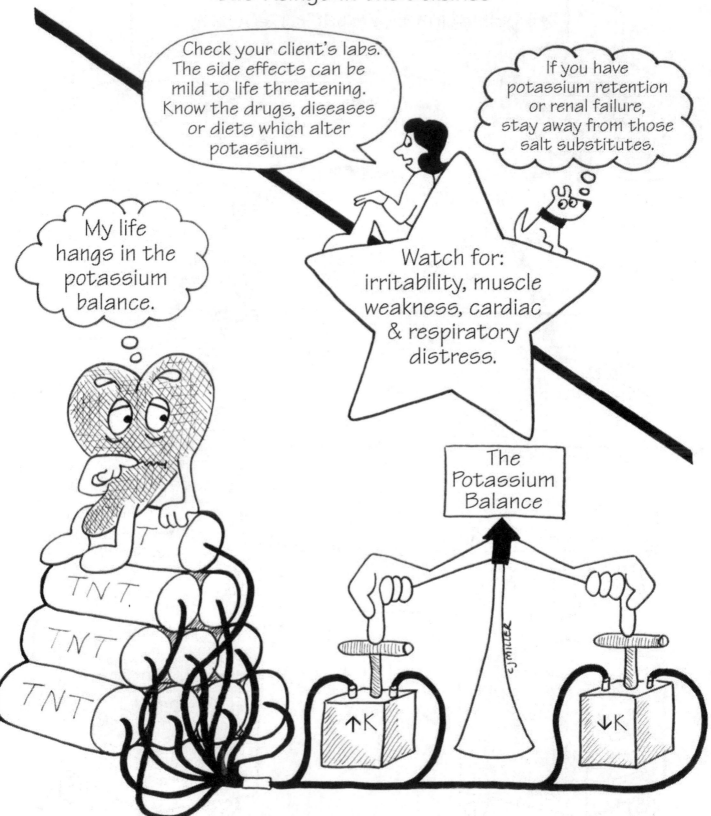

Miscellaneous
Memory Notebook of Nursing: Pharmacology & Diagnostics

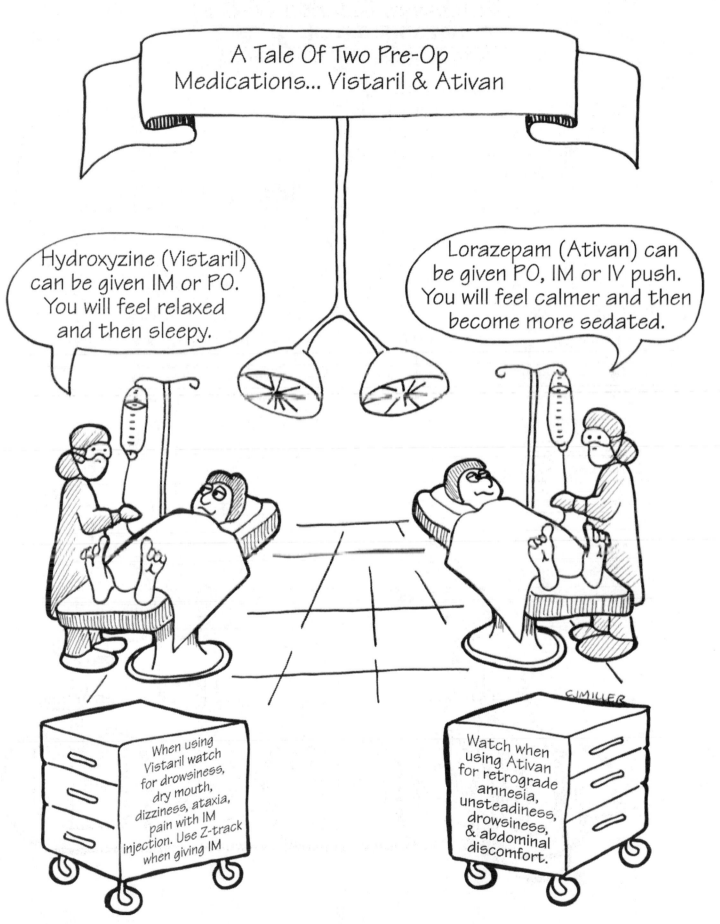

Phenazopyridine (Pyridium)

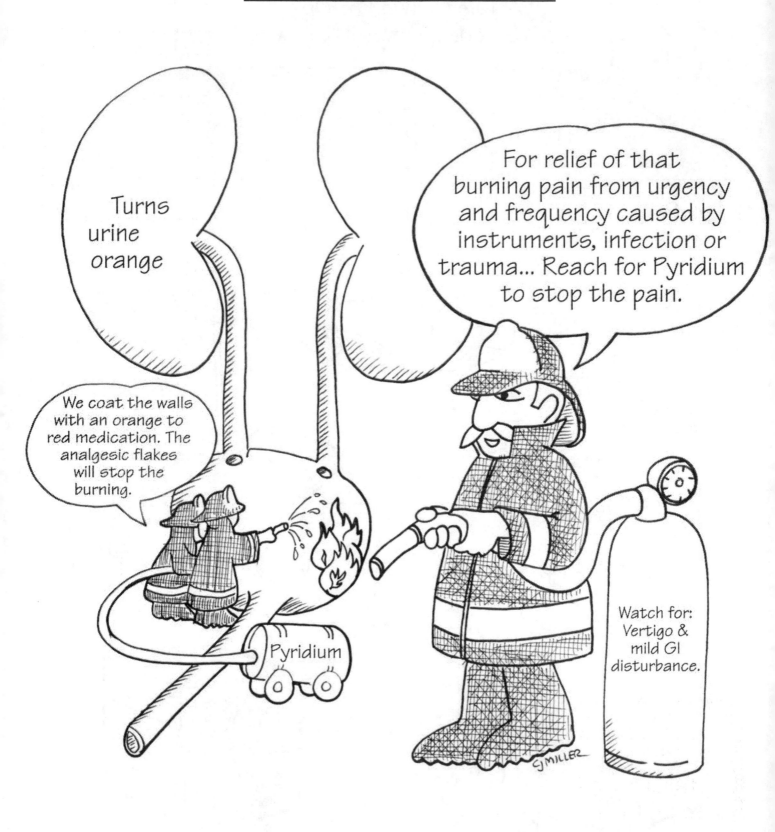

Midazolam (Versed)
Moments Not Remembered

Watch for:
- Respiratory depression
- Arrhythmias
- Hypotension
- Unresponsiveness
- Agitation
- Confusion

Thank goodness for the conscious sedation of Versed. It's moments like these he wouldn't want to remember.

Oh... I think I went too far!

CJMILLER

Use caution with COPD, heart failure, and renal failure.

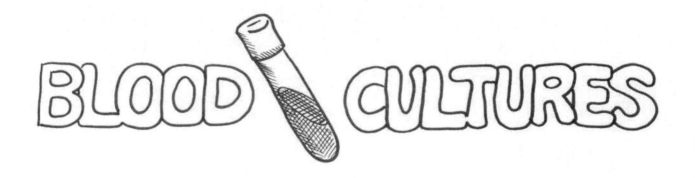

BLOOD CULTURES

☑ Draw when temperature is rising

☑ Collect before starting antibiotics

☑ Clean skin per protocol

☑ Draw 2 cultures 40-60 minutes apart

☑ Collect in appropriate blood collection set

☑ Use 5-10 ml of blood

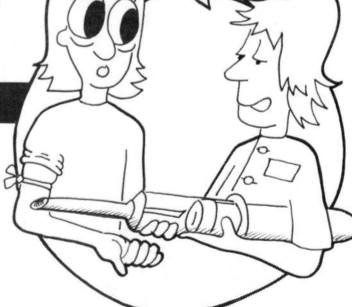

CJMILLER

Laboratory Cultures
Memory Notebook of Nursing: Pharmacology & Diagnostics

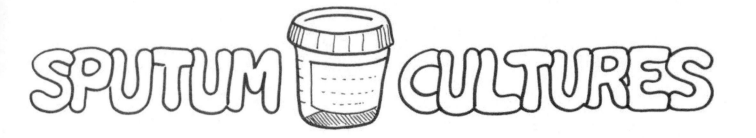

SPUTUM CULTURES

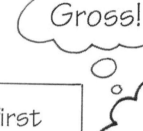

> Gross!

- ☑ Collect sample first thing in the morning
- ☑ Try not to contaminate with saliva or sinus drainage
- ☑ Collect before starting antibiotics

SPUTUM SAMPLE

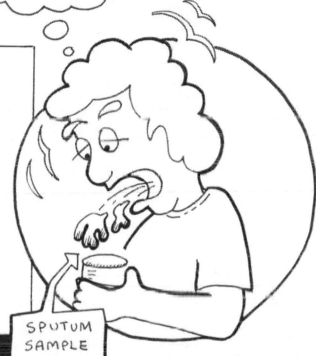

CJMILLER

> If your client is on antibiotics, be sure to write the name of the drug on the slip. As for all labs, label accurately and get to the lab ASAP!

STOOL CULTURES

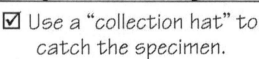

☑ Use a "collection hat" to catch the specimen.

☑ You need about an inch of stool which you or the client can collect using a sterile tongue blade.

☑ Place specimen in a sterile container; try to keep it free from urine.

CJMILLER

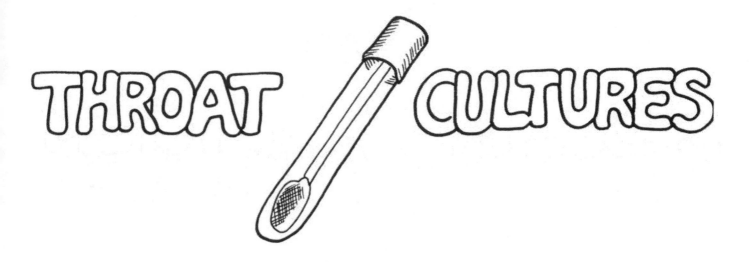

THROAT CULTURES

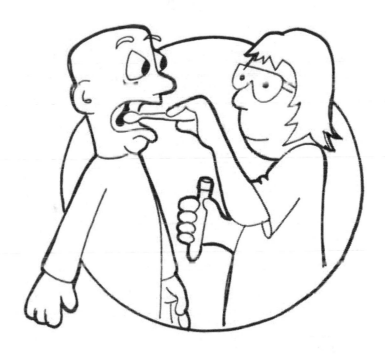

☑ Collect culture prior to starting antibiotics.
☑ Swab the inflammed or ulcerated area of the throat.
☑ Place swab or applicator in culturette tube with it's medium.
☑ If client is on an antibiotic, write the name of the drug on the lab slip.
☑ Label specimen appropriately.

CJMILLER

URINE CULTURES

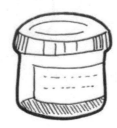

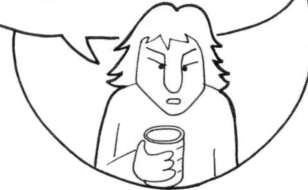

When I do a clean catch or midstream, I must clean the area surrounding the urethra... ...Start midstream, then fill a sterile specimen cup with 5-10ml of urine.

CJMILLER

S. Smith
rm# 303
11-12-04

The initial release of urine flushes the urethra. The test is best done on the first morning voiding and the specimen needs to go to the lab immediately.

Label Accurately!!!!

WOUND 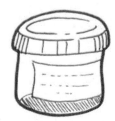 CULTURES

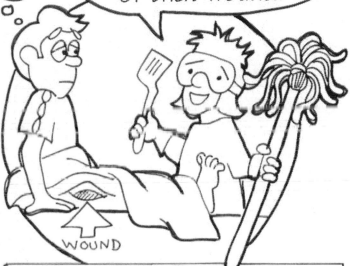

Hold still... I need to get a culture of that wound.

WOUND

Always...
- Use a culture kit or sterile culture tube and cotton swab.
- Remove superficial debris - need a specimen from tissue deep in the wound.
- Gently swab the wound
- Avoid touching swab to intact skin at wound edge.
- Place swab in culture tube.

CJMILLER

Sam Smith, Rm 422 abd wound culture

Sam Smith, Rm 422 abd wound culture

Ammonia Plasma Test

(Adult 15-45 mcg/dl)

Ammonia is a byproduct of protein break down by the liver, which then converts ammonia to urea and excretes it.

Today's Special: <u>Liver</u> with protein products converted to urea

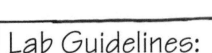

Lab Guidelines:
- Preferrably fasting 8 hours before test (H_2O is okay).
- No smoking for several hours prior to test.
- Draw 5ml of blood in a heparinized tube.
- Get blood to lab on ice.

Drugs that could alter the test are antibiotics, alcohol, potassium salts.

Laboratory Blood Tests
Memory Notebook of Nursing: Pharmacology & Diagnostics
© 2005 Nursing Education
Consultants, Inc.

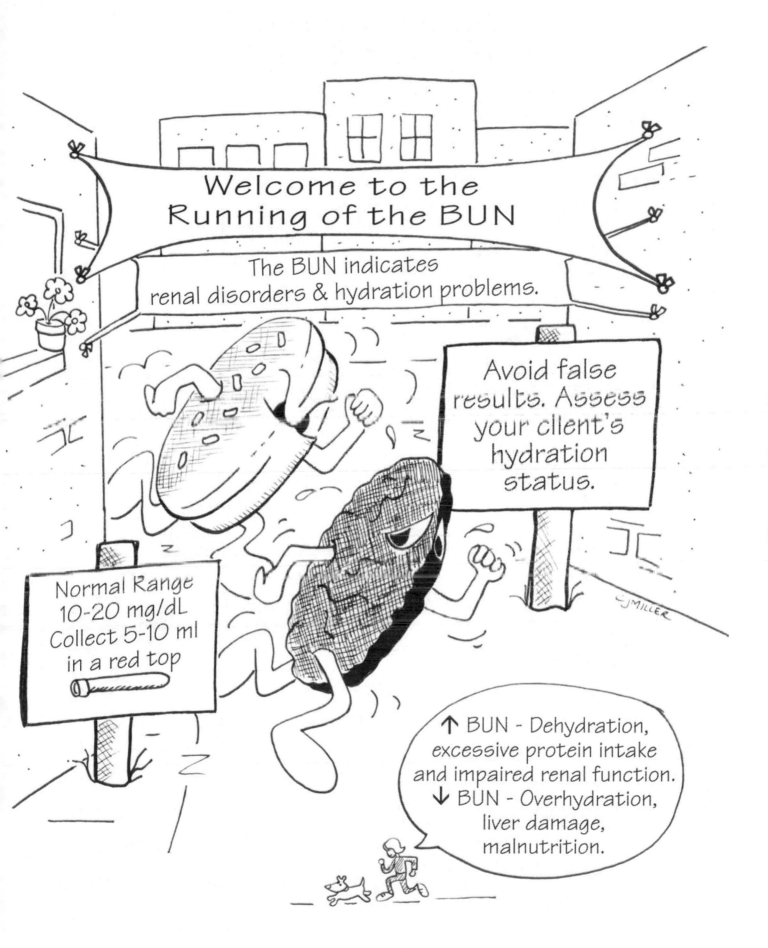

Creatinine and Creatinine Clearance

With renal impairment, serum creatinine goes up, but urinary clearance will go down.

Kidney

Serum
• Creatinine •

Men 0.8 to 1.8 mg/dL
Women 0.5 to 1.5 mg/dL

Increases with kidney malfunction

Urinary
• Creatinine •
Clearance
85 to 135 ml/min
Requires a 24 hour urine specimine. Decreases with renal malfunction

CJMILLER

With unilateral kidney disease, a decrease in creatinine clearance is not expected if the other kidney is healthy

Laboratory Blood Tests
Memory Notebook of Nursing: Pharmacology & Diagnostics

Serum Digoxin Level

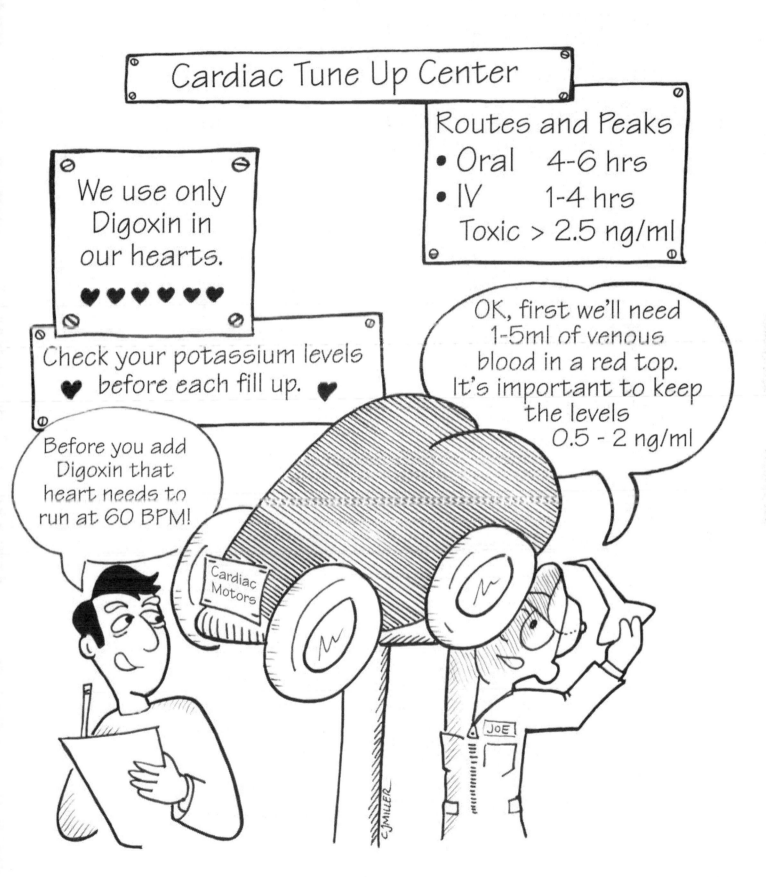

Laboratory Blood Tests
Memory Notebook of Nursing: Pharmacology & Diagnostics

Fibrinogen

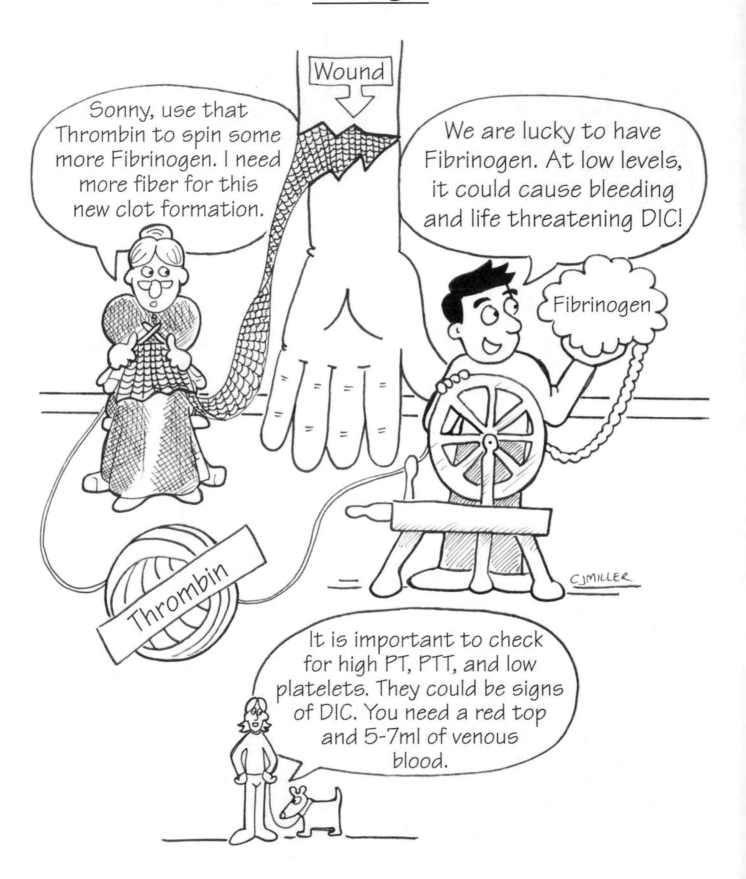

Gamma-Glutamyl Transferase (GGT Serum)

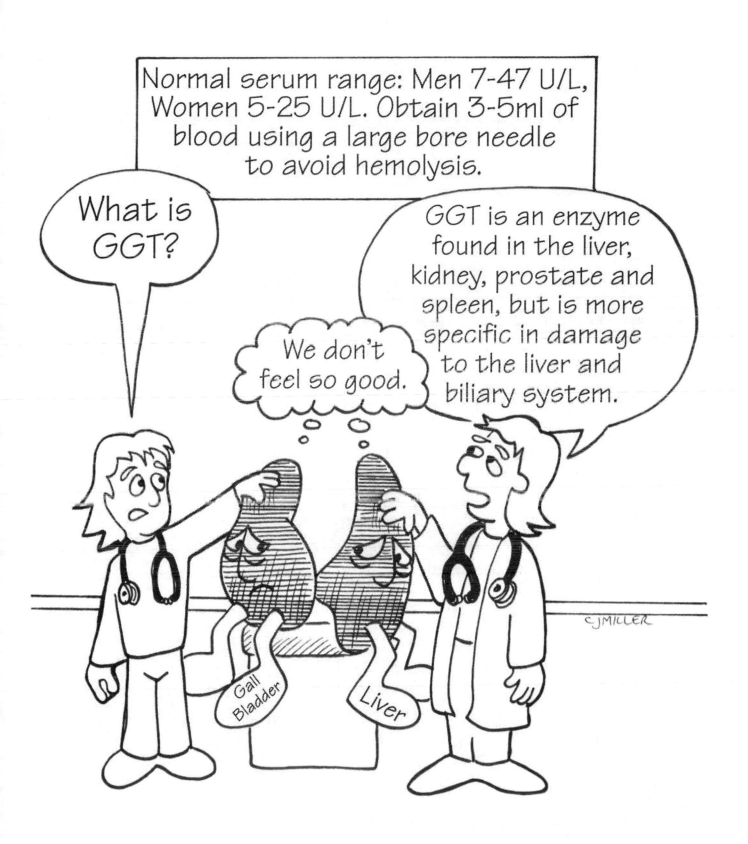

Hematocrit

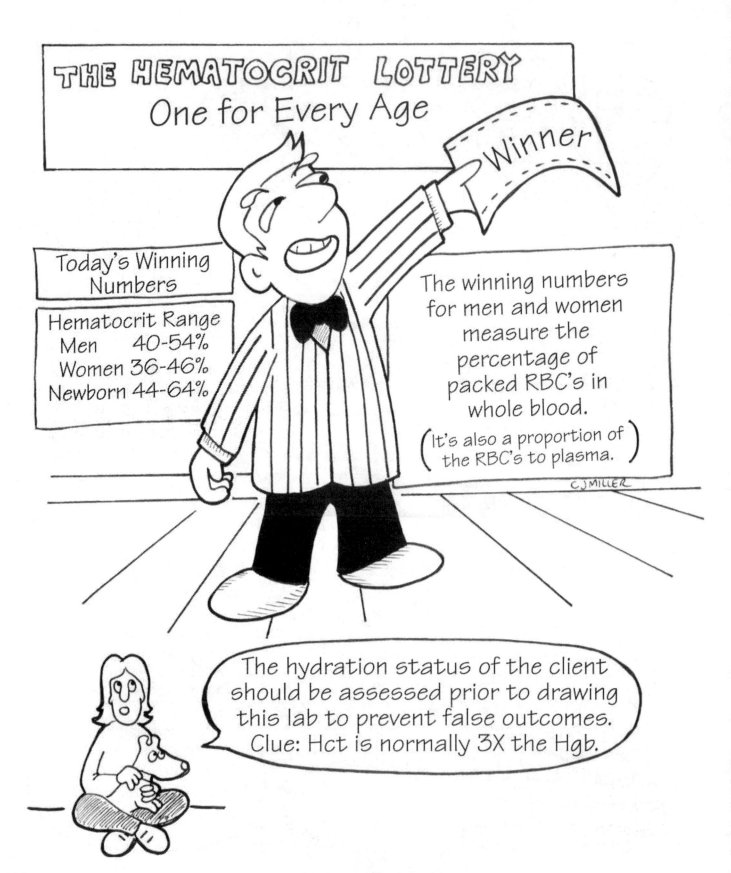

Hemoglobin

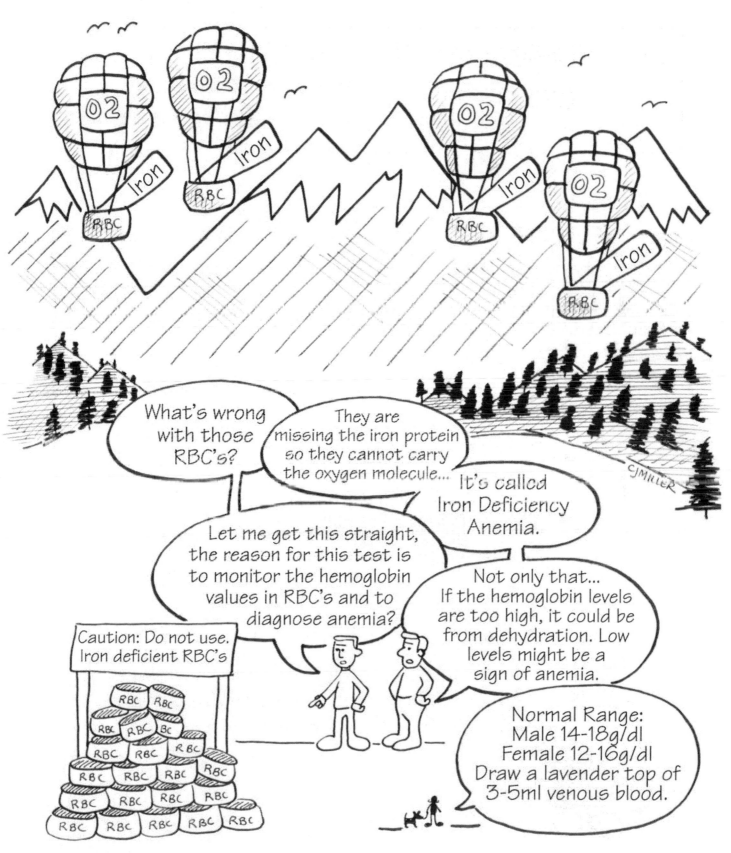

Laboratory Blood Tests
Memory Notebook of Nursing: Pharmacology & Diagnostics

Serum Lipase and Amylase

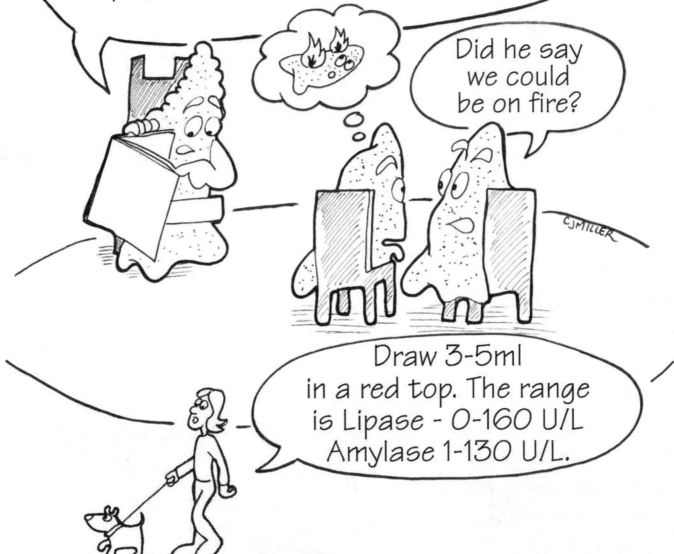

As a pancreas, we release Lipase and Amylase into the blood when we get hurt or inflamed. Both levels rise within 2-12 hours. In 3 days Amylase levels return to normal, but Lipase stays elevated for up to 7 to 10 days, helping in late diagnosis of pancreatitis.

Did he say we could be on fire?

Draw 3-5ml in a red top. The range is Lipase - 0-160 U/L Amylase 1-130 U/L.

Lipoproteins

If It Tastes Good, It's Probably Bad For You!

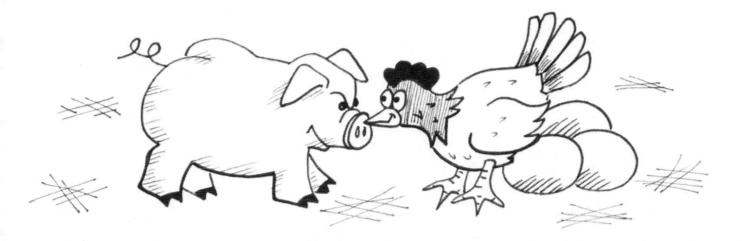

Low Density Lipoproteins...

(>130mg/dl) increases risk of development of coronary artery disease.

High Density Lipoproteins...

(>60mg/dl) are Good For You

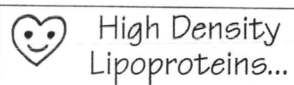

Warning: This is a 12 to 14 hour fast (except water) and no alcoholic beverages for 24 hours before test. Draw 5-7ml in Red Top

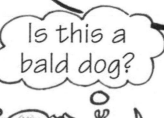

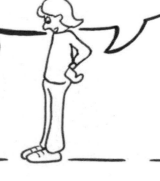

Serum Sodium and Chloride

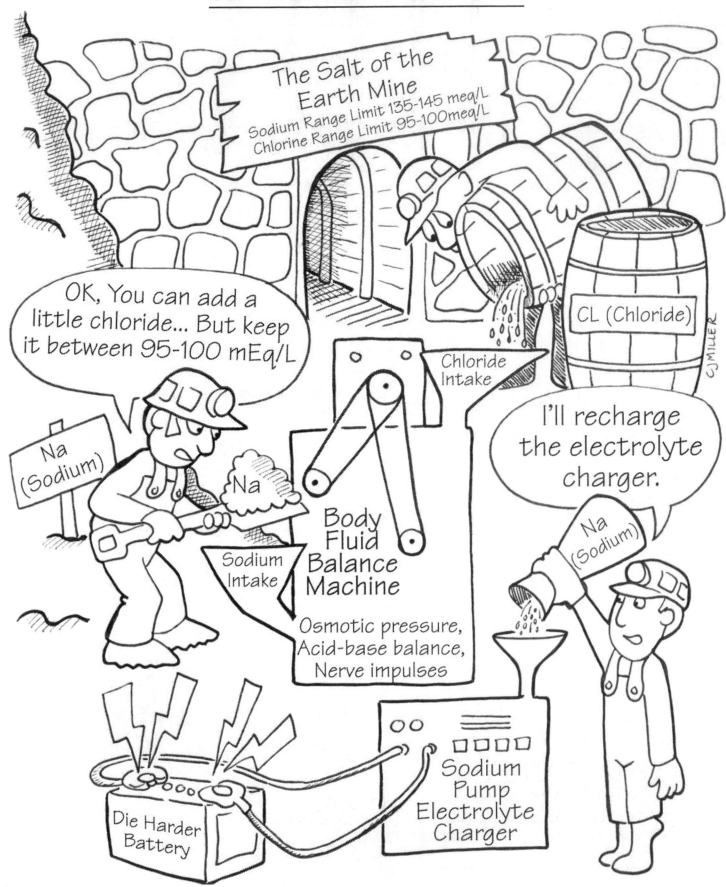

Laboratory Blood Tests
Memory Notebook of Nursing: Pharmacology & Diagnostics

PTT and APTT

"A Time and Place To Bleed"

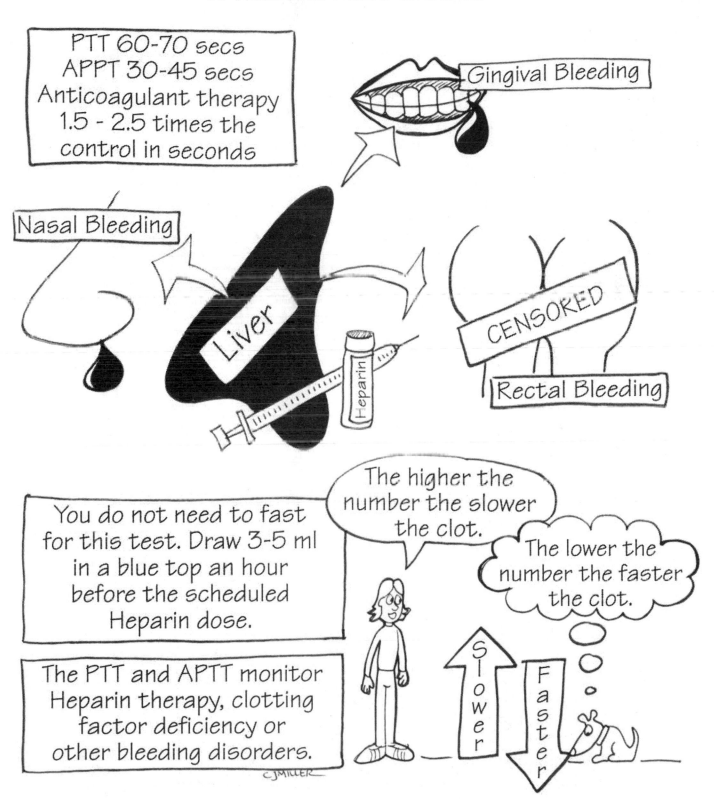

PTT 60-70 secs
APPT 30-45 secs
Anticoagulant therapy
1.5 - 2.5 times the
control in seconds

Gingival Bleeding

Nasal Bleeding

Liver

Heparin

CENSORED

Rectal Bleeding

You do not need to fast
for this test. Draw 3-5 ml
in a blue top an hour
before the scheduled
Heparin dose.

The PTT and APTT monitor
Heparin therapy, clotting
factor deficiency or
other bleeding disorders.

The higher the
number the slower
the clot.

The lower the
number the faster
the clot.

Slower

Faster

C.J.MILLER

Mean Platelet Value (MPV)

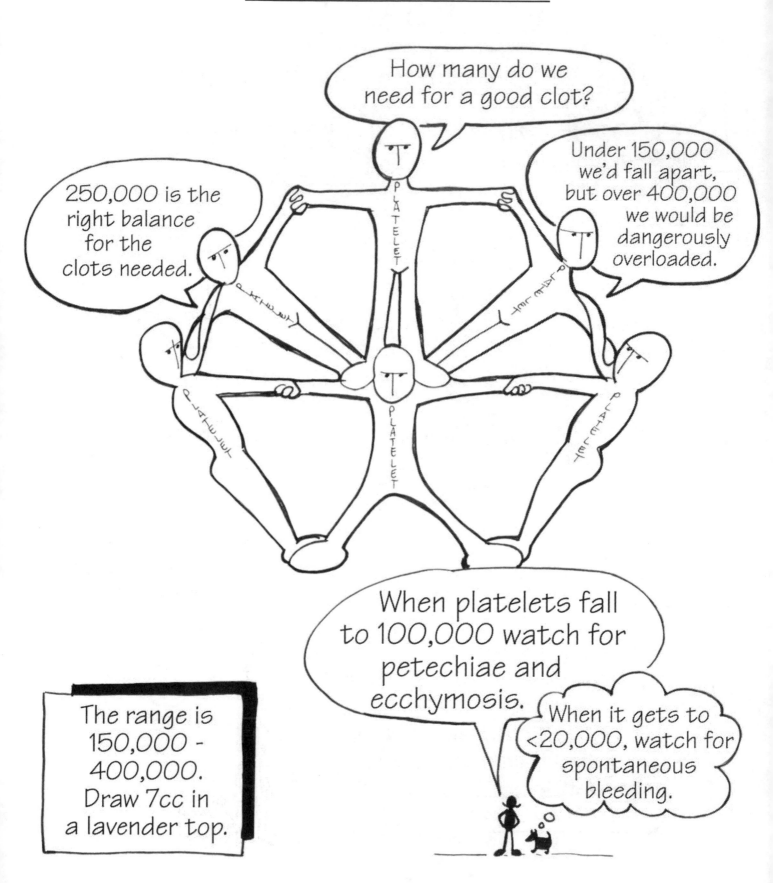

Potassium (Serum)

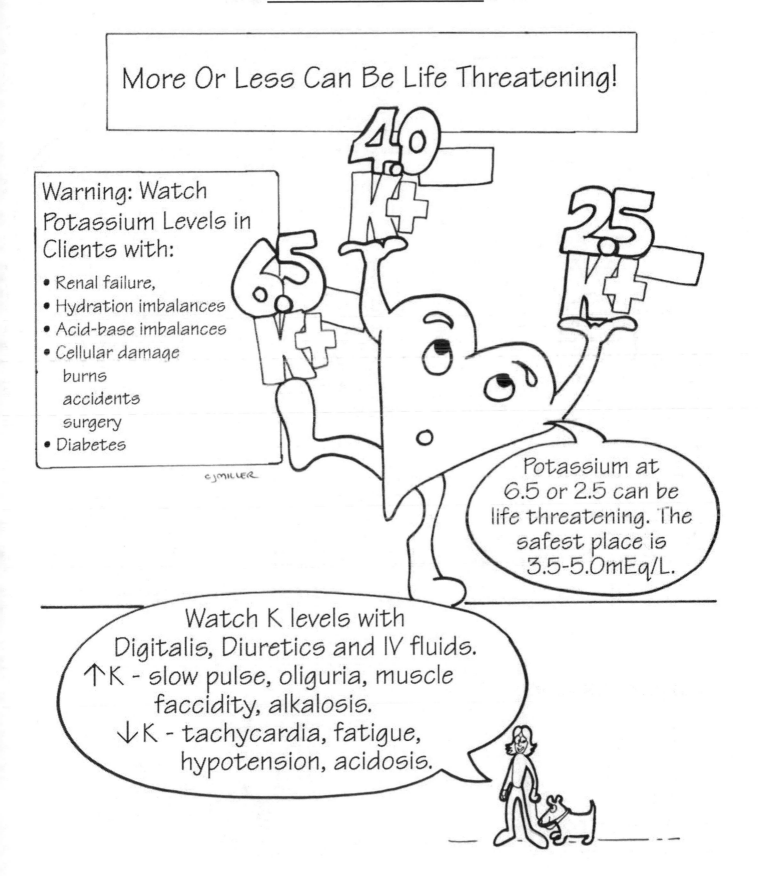

More Or Less Can Be Life Threatening!

Warning: Watch Potassium Levels in Clients with:

- Renal failure,
- Hydration imbalances
- Acid-base imbalances
- Cellular damage
  burns
  accidents
  surgery
- Diabetes

CJMILLER

4.0 K+

6.5 K+

2.5 K+

Potassium at 6.5 or 2.5 can be life threatening. The safest place is 3.5-5.0mEq/L.

Watch K levels with Digitalis, Diuretics and IV fluids.
↑K - slow pulse, oliguria, muscle faccidity, alkalosis.
↓K - tachycardia, fatigue, hypotension, acidosis.

Prothrombin Time (PT) and INR

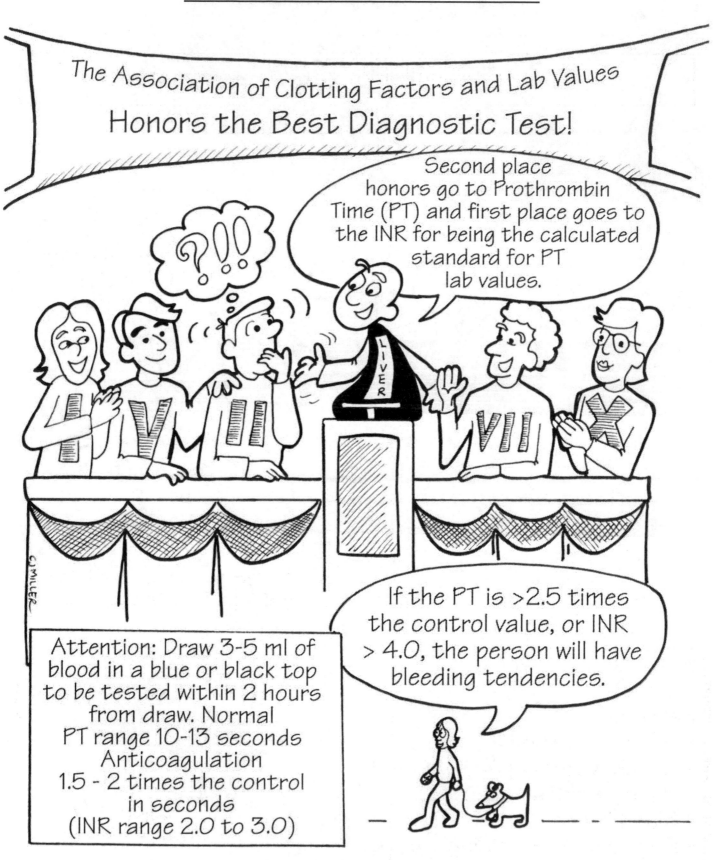

Prostate Specific Antigen (PSA)

It's a guy thing for those with a prostate.

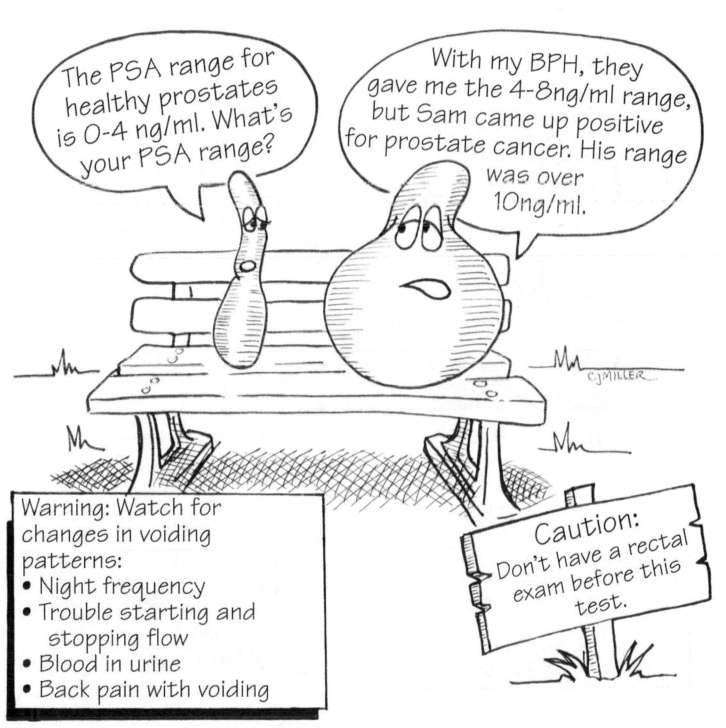

T (Toxoplasmosis)
O (Other-usually Syphilis)
R (Rubella)
C (Cytomegalovirus - CMV)
H (Herpes Simplex - HSV)

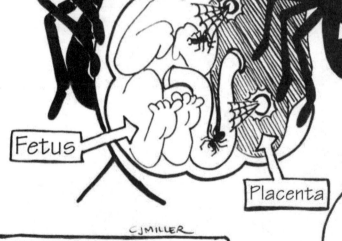

We cause the worst damage during the first trimester.

By crossing the placenta we can cause congenital malformations, abortions or stillborns.

Fetus

Placenta

You need 7ml of blood in a red top

Reference values measured in IgG and IgM titer antibodies. A negative show is the best news.

CJMILLER

Laboratory Blood Tests
Memory Notebook of Nursing: Pharmacology & Diagnostics

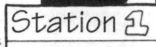

White Blood Cells (WBC) Total

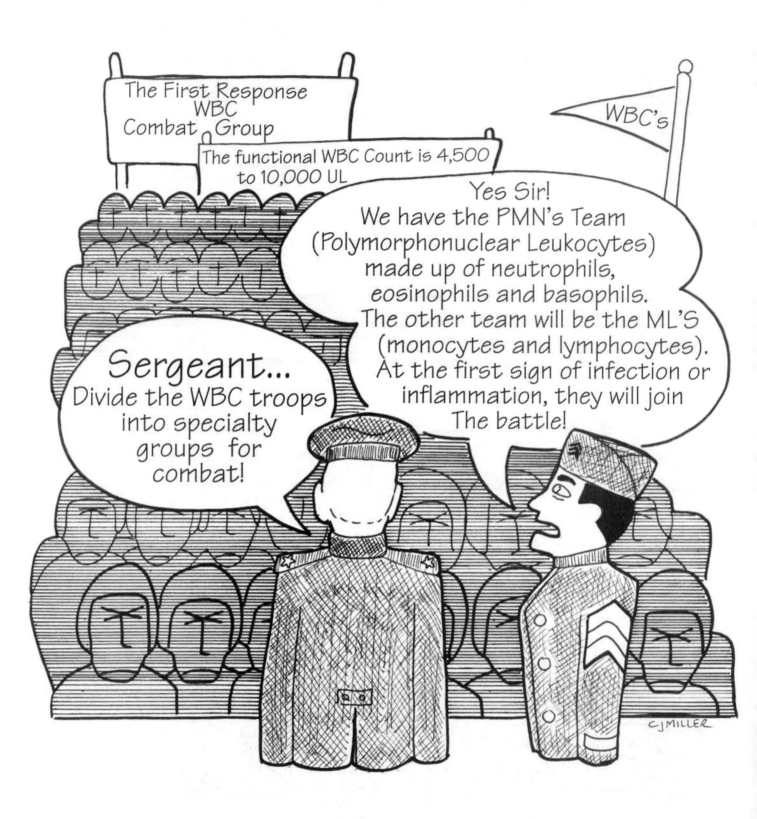

Bone Densitometry (Bone Mineral Density)

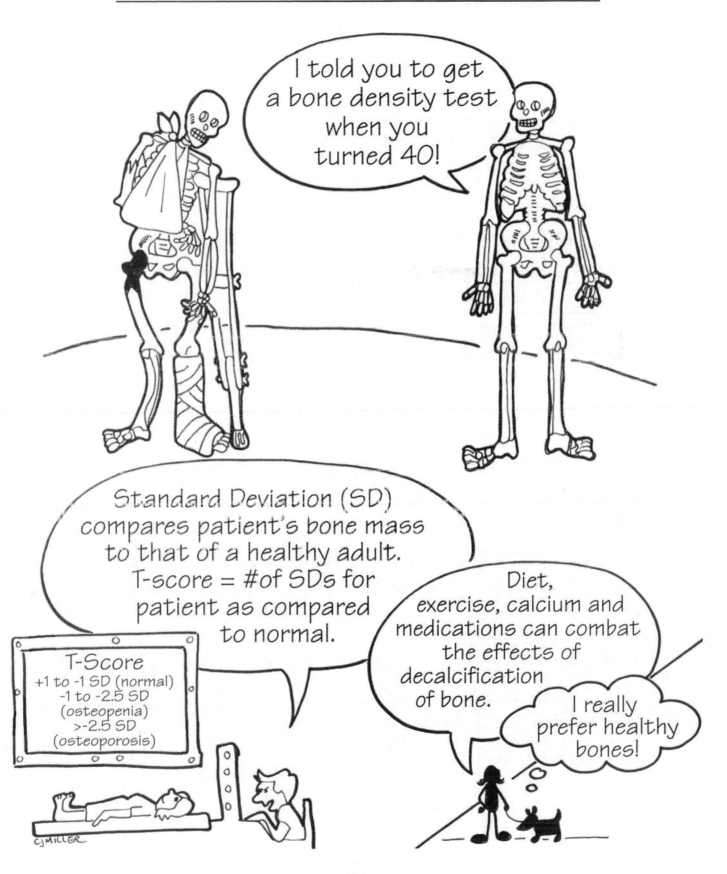

© 2005 Nursing Education
Consultants, Inc.

Memory Notebook of Nursing: Pharmacology & Diagnostics

Bronchoscopy

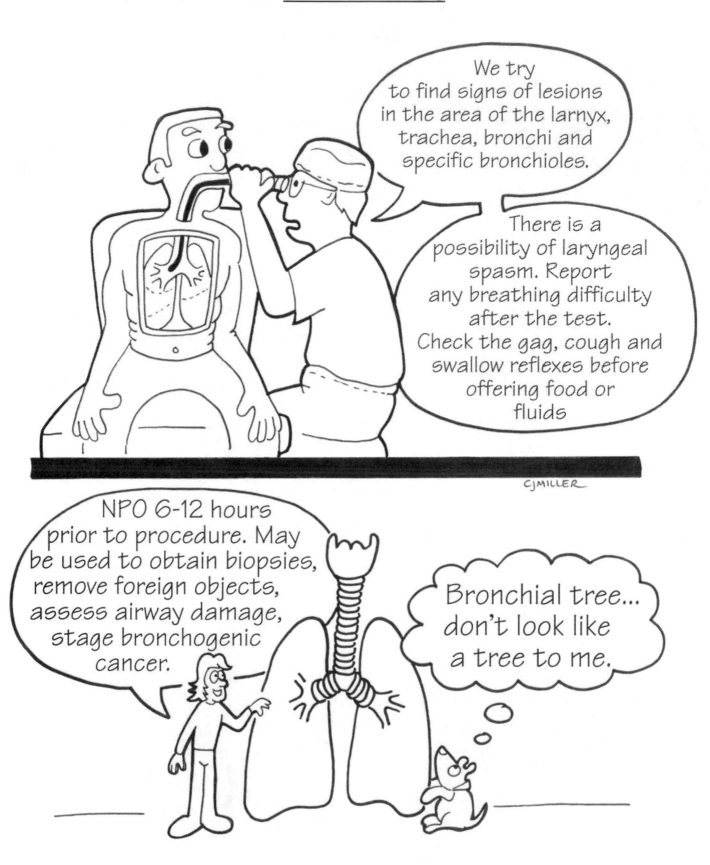

Diagnostic Tests
Memory Notebook of Nursing: Pharmacology & Diagnostics

Chorionic Villi Biopsy (CVB)

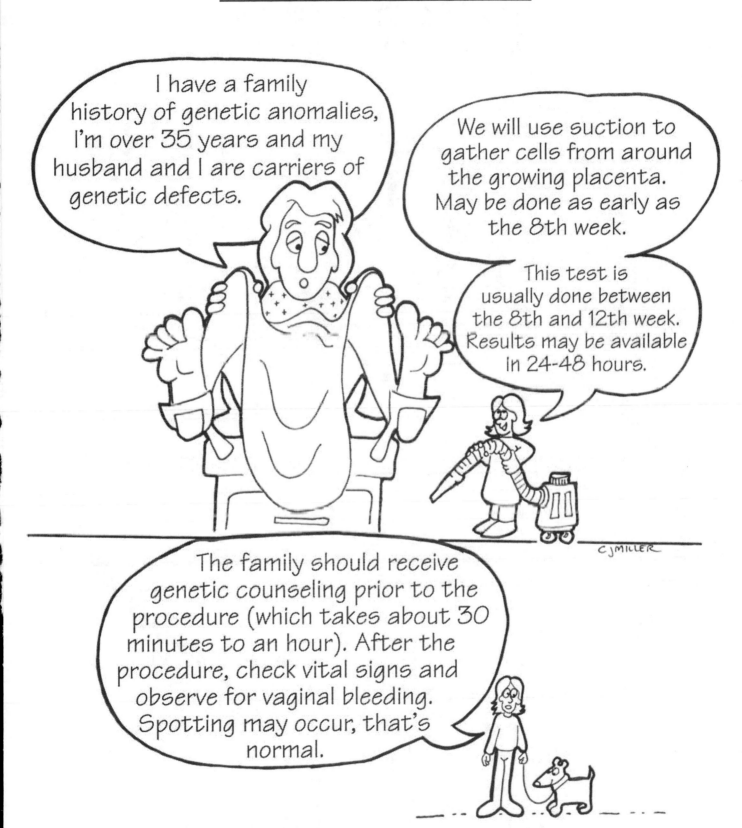

Master Guaiac's "Occult Blood Now!"

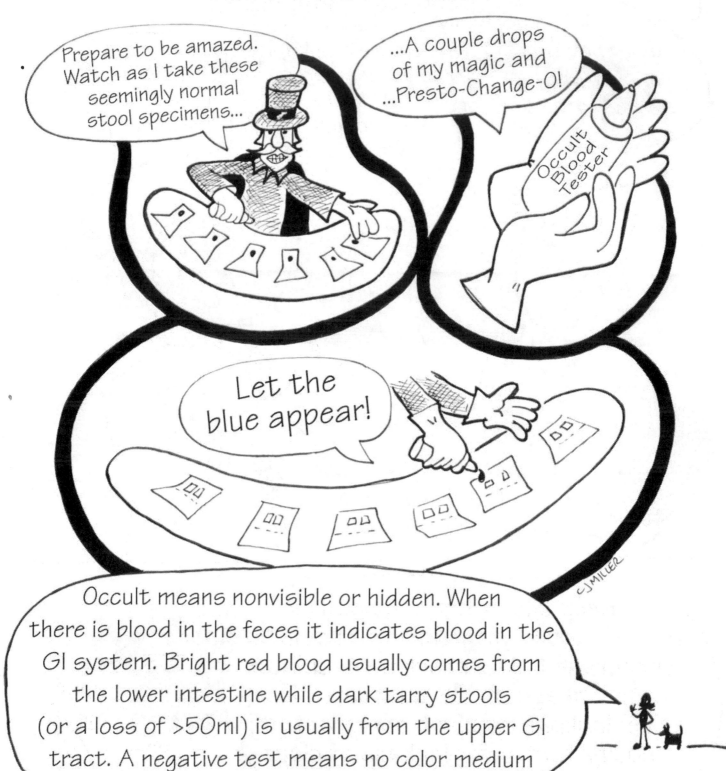

Prepare to be amazed. Watch as I take these seemingly normal stool specimens...

...A couple drops of my magic and ...Presto-Change-O!

Occult Blood Tester

Let the blue appear!

Occult means nonvisible or hidden. When there is blood in the feces it indicates blood in the GI system. Bright red blood usually comes from the lower intestine while dark tarry stools (or a loss of >50ml) is usually from the upper GI tract. A negative test means no color medium seen in stool.

Spinal Fluid Analysis

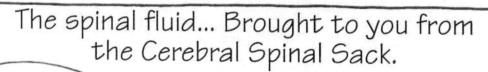

The spinal fluid... Brought to you from the Cerebral Spinal Sack.

What will you look for?

We'll look for the color to be clear, pressure 90-180cm H_2O, protein 15-45mg/dL, glucose 40/70mg/dL, minimal WBC's and the presence of bacteria.

CJMILLER

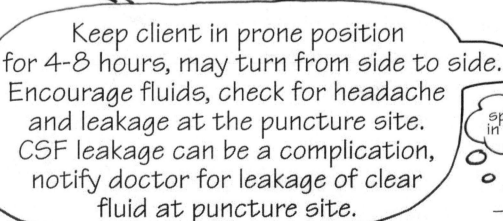

Keep client in prone position for 4-8 hours, may turn from side to side. Encourage fluids, check for headache and leakage at the puncture site. CSF leakage can be a complication, notify doctor for leakage of clear fluid at puncture site.

Label specimens in the order drawn.

ACUTE CEREBRAL OVERLOAD SYNDROME
AS RELATED TO I.D.S.D. (IMMINENT DEADLINE STRESS DISORDER)

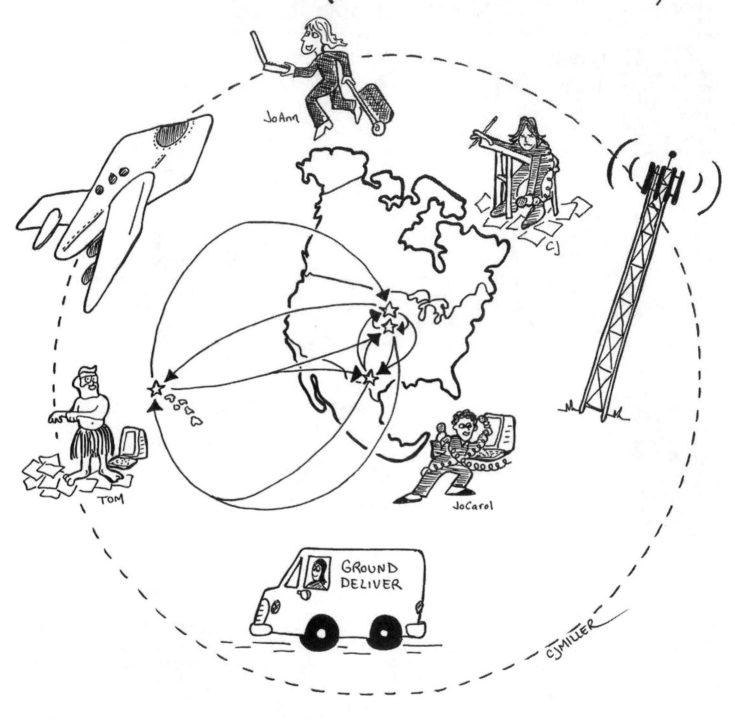

Index